DEREK WRIGHT

MY STORY IN BLACK AND WHITE

Four decades Fixing the Mags

WITH JOHN WRIGHT

First published by Pitch Publishing, 2024

Pitch Publishing
9 Donnington Park,
85 Birdham Road,
Chichester,
West Sussex,
PO20 7AJ
www.pitchpublishing.co.uk
info@pitchpublishing.co.uk

ISBN 978 1 80150 742 4

Printed and bound in the UK on FSC® certified paper in line
with our continuing commitment to ethical business practices,
sustainability and the environment.

Typesetting and origination by Pitch Publishing

Printed and bound by CPI Anthony Rowe, UK

Kevin Keegan

Derek was an incredibly loyal member of staff at NUFC for so many years.

No one is irreplaceable but he just might be!

Alan Shearer

Del Boy is the nicest of men, a touch of class and a gentleman. He was a highly trusted member of staff with great experience and knowledge of players' needs. To add to that he's undoubtedly a brilliant physio.

Stuart Pearce

I was fortunate enough to join Newcastle United in 1997 and lucky enough to have Derek as my physio. We became good friends.

My defining memory of Degs is his enormous appetite and his love of music, which both combined one night at a Stranglers gig in York, both eating and drinking to excess and finishing the night pogoing with the big man for the duration of the gig.

As U21 manager I asked Degs to join my staff as I knew that his professionalism and patriotism would be a great fit, not to mention his loyalty.

What a Man!!!

Degs – I I love you

Contents

Glossary of Geordie and Colloquial Words

bairn	child
bogey	homemade go-cart
bonty	bonfire
cadge	borrow
clammin'	hungry
clarts	mud
crack	Anglo version of craic
divvent	don't
gan	go
hacky	dirty
hoy	throw
hyem	home
marra	friend
mek	make
muckle	big and strong
napper	head
nee	no
nivvor	never
nor	no
nowt	nothing
oot	out
parched	thirsty
pagga	to hit
paggad	exhausted
radgie	crazy
ruction	disturbance
scrag	ruffle, make a mess
stott	hit, bounce
stotty	bread
telt	told
welly	kick hard
whey	well
wor	our

Chapter 1

Arsenal

'GEORDIE, MAN! Gis a hand with me bogey. The rope's knackin' me hand.' I showed my friend my blistered palm.

'Oh, shite,' he replied, grabbing a share of the loop of hemp rope I was holding. We were walking down the steep hill from Stanley towards my home in South Stanley. On the homemade go-cart were the contents of a hundredweight bag of coal, carefully divided into ten paper bags from the original hessian sack; the contents were now spilling on to the path every time the cart's wheels went over a divot. I was in big trouble: that coal should have been fish and chips.

My aspirations of being a business entrepreneur ended that day as a 12-year-old lad in the fading light of a 1971 summer's evening. Unfortunately for me, the cost of a bag of coal was just a bit less than the pound note my dad had given me for fish and chips 'four-times', which lit the 'stupid' lightbulb in my head. Mam and Dad had sent me up the one-mile hill to Kaiser's chip shop for a rare family treat. George and I should have been there for the chippy opening at six o'clock, but we decided to pop into the shop next door first. That's where we spotted the sacks of coal for sale, 75p a bag. I came up with the bright idea of dividing the contents and becoming Stanley's youngest and most brilliant-ever

9

coal merchant, roaming door to door to visit our eager customers. Selling ten bags for 10p each meant we would make 25p profit and still get the fish and chips! We cadged some paper bags from the shop owner and gleefully started our enterprise. By the time the bags were ready, stacked neatly on the bogey outside the chippy, we were already filthy with coal dust.

Of course, no one in the houses along Spen Street was interested in buying ripped paper bags of coal from two dirty imps. Time passed and the implications slowly dawned: ten bags of coal, spilling out of the tattered paper, no fish and chips, sun starting to set. Eventually the march of time forced a decision and we had to head back. First, I pulled the go-cart, but as the hill steepened the cart pulled me by the hand down the hill.

'Me da's ganna kill us, Geordie.'

'Mine win't. He doesn't care when I get hyem.'

'Whey, mine does.' George looked at me with his hacky face and shrugged. *His* dad *didn't* care. Of course, both of my parents were panicking by this stage. In the 1970s there was a considerable amount of flexibility about staying out, but being absent four hours late, in the dark, was beyond the pale. When Dad finally saw me, he showed his relief by greeting his errant son with a kick up the arse. Ironically, I fell into the full coal bunker outside the house. Of course, he blamed it on us returning minus fish and chips and money, with a bogey full of coal. My mother managed to calm him down and ran a bath for me to clean myself up. She explained that my dad had been in a panic, frantically searching the streets. A bit of TLC from Mam was what I needed and everything after that was right as rain.

* * *

I was born on 10 October 1958. I grew up on the streets of Stanley in County Durham. The town was in the process of closing the pits but back then it was still very much a mining community. My first school was South Moor Greenland Primary School, where many years later they filmed some of Martin Shaw's *Inspector George Gently* series. I met three boys on my first day: Alan Reay, Geoff Hind and Alan Reader. Sixty years later and I still see them regularly.

My parents had to share my granddad's house on Elm Street in South Moor; my brother and I shared a bedroom with our parents for four years until a council house became available. The place we moved to was Chiltern Gardens in South Stanley, about two miles away. The estate would be described in modern terms as a 'sink estate', a place to put antisocial tenants. Many of the residents did have significant social problems and there was a lot of crime, not that I was aware of that at the time. Growing up, we were oblivious to that, it was all we knew. I do remember once my dad carefully planted a large privet hedge around our garden on the end terrace, only to discover two hours later that it had all been moved and planted in a garden up the street (retrieved by my irate father with a threat of violence to the perpetrator's father).

In hindsight, a wide and eclectic social mix lived on our street. Beautifully manicured gardens maintained by elderly couples or plots bursting with expertly grown fruits and vegetables owned by tradesmen would be separated by desolate yards full of detritus such as cushionless settees or damp mattresses surrounded by nettles and dock. One family at the top of the street had even ripped up half of their floorboards to put on the fire. Stray dogs constantly roamed the streets, harassing the children. We would occasionally crowd around two dogs 'stuck together by the tail', waiting for one of the mothers to come out of the house wearing the ubiquitous pinny carrying a basin of water and throw it over the dogs.

In many ways it was a blessed childhood. My brother John and I had loving parents, Pat and Derek. We lived in an environment full of adventure. Our house was on the end of a terrace that was beside farm fields and beyond that were two woods, thoughtfully named First and Second Wood. When not in school, my childhood involved many hours roaming through the fields and woods, covering huge distances, probably some 20 square miles. We would be out all day, climbing trees looking for birds' nests, or fishing sticklebacks out of the ponds, or raiding fat, green gooseberries and rhubarb from gardens. Sometimes on Sundays we would spy on the miners playing pitch and toss in the heart of Second Wood, standing by an old poplar tree called the 'Witchy'. We saw them scatter once when the 'polis' drove down the path towards them, running here and there in their pinstriped suits and cloth caps.

It was a great time for street games such as cannon (tin cans with sticks on hit by tennis balls), tally-ho (defend your base against the marauding hordes) and montakitty (a version of leap-frog: 'Montakitty, montakitty one, two, three; finger, thumb or little ganny?'). We also made 'javelins' out of bamboo sticks that we sharpened and feathered, launching them hundreds of feet with nothing more than a knotted piece of string. October was always the most exciting time as we prepared for bonfire night. Boys (and girls) from different streets would build their own bonfires and would spend the evenings going 'bonty-raiding' other gangs' stashes of wood. I'm ashamed to confess that we would occasionally go down the wood and fell a tree for the centre-pole of the bonty, too. Other childhood memories include a rag-and-bone man called 'Dingly' Bell with his horse and cart, French onion sellers wheeling their bicycles up and down the streets, wearing Breton shirts and berets, and wedding 'chuck-outs' or 'hoy-oots', when the bride-to-be would throw loose change out of her car on the way to church, with all of us 'bairns' charging around after the car picking up pennies, thruppences and tanners.

One of my favourite games was 'gates'. In our street, two rows of houses faced each other, with a single road running up to a cul-de-sac at the top of the road. Each front garden had a gate that we opened and used as a goal. About six of us would defend our own goal while everyone tried to score in everyone else's goal. Once you let in, say, five or ten goals, you were out. The one defending the goal conceding the fewest was the winner. As a shout-out to women's football, by far the best player in the street was a girl called Eunice Petrie. Unfortunately, in those days there was no option of playing amateur football, let alone professionally, for women; if it was, she would have made it.

It was about the time of the fish and chips incident that I was starting to realise I could play football. I'd already made it into the Greenland junior school team, first as goalkeeper but then as centre-half. We'd won the Stanley League and the Newcastle player and legend Frank Clark presented us with the trophy. It was after moving to Tanfield Grammar School to the north of the town that I started showing greater promise. Physically I developed early, and I was blessed with speed, winning awards for sprinting at the Durham County schools' athletics competitions. I was also stronger than my peers, and fearless, meaning I progressed to representing Stanley District and then county for Durham schools. That was in the days when Sunderland and Gateshead were still part of the county.

My parents came to games when possible. My father is an intelligent guy, but he left school at 14 without any qualifications to his name. That's what nearly all working-class children did then. After completing National Service, he finished a six-year boilermaker's apprenticeship at Redheugh Iron and Steel Company on the Tyne and became a welder. We hardly saw him because of the hours plus overtime he worked. He would be up and out the house in the morning before we were up. He had to walk the mile or so up the hill to Stanley and then get the bus to Gateshead. If he wasn't doing overtime, he would arrive back in the street in the early evening. He would stand and watch our game of gates, giving encouragement and advice, before going in the house to see Mam. She had a better education than him and went to Stanley Grammar. Unfortunately, falling pregnant with me out of wedlock and then giving birth while she was only 19 meant the end to her studies for the time. She'd completed training as a radiographer but had to give this employment up when she was expecting John so that she could firstly avoid the radiation risk and then look after the two of us. She became a primary school teacher some years later.

One thing about where I grew up, we were never far from trouble, be it the many intimidating stray dogs let out of the houses by their owners for the day, or other children looking for a fight. I was never impulsively aggressive in that way, but because of a macho culture and the frequency of fights I was immersed in, I discovered I was good at it. I learned that a major factor behind being able to win a street fight was the ability to take pain, as well as meting out whatever damage you could inflict on your opponent. This pain tolerance was something I'd inherited from my dad, which he 'got' in turn from his father, Joseph. Joe was a miner in the Craghead Colliery, but he was also an amateur bare-knuckle boxer. For a while the fighting got out of hand and lads would travel for miles just to 'have a go' at me. I wasn't hard to find, with my bright red hair. I was taught a lesson one day playing gates when I refused to stop our game for the bin wagon and lost a fight with one of the men. Well, a 12-year-old against a fella in his 20s, what would you expect?

I was always calm but determined on the football pitch and, by the age of 13, professional clubs had noticed me. I was approached by several First and Second Division clubs, including Manchester United, Leeds, Liverpool and Birmingham. The two local clubs, Newcastle and Sunderland, were also showing an interest. Stanley's support is split between the two local clubs. It's roughly equal distances between the Stanley and the two cities and therefore the town is split approximately 50:50 for support, at least it was then. Legend has it that a train line ran from the north of the town to Newcastle, and another ran from the south of the town to Sunderland. My dad, always a Newcastle supporter, had 11 siblings and the brothers' support for the two clubs was split.

When I was old enough to go without a grown-up, I went with my Stanley mates to St James' Park when I could. Because I was playing so much football, this meant it was only the occasional weekend match or, more often, a midweek one. I would usually go with Stephen McPhail. We always went in the Leazes End. I remember the blokes selling bags of peanuts. We would hoy down a tanner and they would chuck the bag of peanuts straight back to us.

I particularly remember the Fairs Cup players, especially Wyn Davies, Frank Clark and Pop Robson, and then shortly after that John Tudor and Supermac himself, Malcolm Macdonald. Those who were at his home debut on 21 August 1971 when he scored a hat-trick in the 3-2 win against Liverpool will never forget it. I also have an image in my mind of Alan Foggon on another occasion standing in a centre circle devoid of grass and up to his ankles in clarts.

Like many aspiring professionals, most of my football experience at the time was involved in playing the game, not watching it. With the interest of the two local clubs, it might seem strange that I chose to sign as a schoolboy for Arsenal. The north

London club went to great efforts to court me. I was playing for Stanley Boys up at Consett's Belle Vue Park one freezing afternoon towards the end of 1972 when my dad was approached by a small gentleman wearing a raincoat and trilby. It turned out to be the Arsenal manager, Bertie Mee! The man who had managed Arsenal to the FA Cup and league double win at the end of the previous season had made the effort to travel by train from London just to watch me play. His interest had been sparked by their North East scout, George Emmerson. My parents were impressed by the effort made by Arsenal and when I went down to visit the club their staff, including the chief scout Gordon Clark, were equally professional and welcoming. There was no doubt the whole club had an air of regal quality about it. It's impossible to forget the majestic white Marble Halls at the entrance to Highbury.

So, although I visited other clubs, I'd already made the decision that I wanted to play professional football for Arsenal FC. My parents were invited down with my brother and me. We stayed in the best hotels and were given tickets for shows in the West End. Bertie even made the effort to take my family to restaurants. Before those trips my parents hadn't been on a train or airplane. Their holidays consisted of day trips to South Shields. One evening we were in a swanky restaurant and my dad was offered a liqueur by the maître d'. He requested a lager. The waiter was halfway through reprimanding my dad for such an uncouth request when Mr Mee raised his hand and told him: 'Make that two.'

Over the next year I continued to improve as a player. One notable achievement during that time was that I was part of the Durham Boys County team that won the Northern School Counties Championship at Roker Park. Other now familiar lads I played with at the time were Derek Scott, who went to play for Burnley and Bolton over 400 times, and Stan Cummins, the

Middlesbrough and Sunderland forward. When we won the cup we were presented with the trophy by the Sunderland manager, Bob Stokoe, less than a week after he'd run on to the pitch in his cream-coloured raincoat following their famous FA Cup victory. Toon historians will know that Bob was an important ex-Newcastle United player, not just our rivals' manager: he'd played for us for a decade and was in the 1955 FA Cup-winning team.

I was also brought under the umbrella of potential England Schoolboys and was invited to an instructional course held by the FA; I then signed as an associated schoolboy with Arsenal on 6 September 1973 at the age of 14. Shortly after my 15th birthday I went for England trials in Leeds but was ultimately unsuccessful. That didn't deter me and for the remainder of that academic year and the next I continued to improve as a footballer. I travelled regularly to north London. Most Friday afternoons, after school, a taxi arrived at our house in Stanley and drove me to Central Station. I would get the train to King's Cross to be met by the chief scout, Gordon Clark, or his assistant Ernie Collett. They would always be waiting for me without fail, even when the train was hours late. They would then make sure I got to my digs. Our youth team played in the South East Counties League. I would make the reverse trip home on Sunday afternoon and arrive back in the evening to be ready for school the following morning.

It was around this time that my dad lost his job. He'd been forced to move downriver to Ryton Marine on the Newcastle side of the Tyne as some of the shipyards started to close, but eventually that place suffered the same demise. They blamed it on Japanese and South Korean shipyards undercutting the UK shipyards' prices. Whatever the reason, he was on the dole with no prospect or work. This was the time of recession, inflation and the Three-Day Week. There was mass unemployment and, to add insult to injury, he'd worked the last six months prior to being sacked for no wages.

The situation where we lived in Stanley worsened as well. There were always some chronically unemployed men on the estate, but the numbers out of work continued to rise. Many of the children were feral. I didn't see much of my brother John at the time, but I knew he was spending more and more time in the 'wrong crowd'. Two of these lads eventually progressed years later to being imprisoned for being professional birds' eggs thieves. The situation culminated in John getting into trouble with the police. Fortunately for him, we moved house because my parents could finally afford a mortgage. My dad and two of his foreman work colleagues had been approached by three of the ex-managers of Ryton Marine to see if they were interested in starting a metal fabrication business. The three tradesmen had been hand-picked by the managers for their known work ethic and ability. So, the increased income from their fledgling business in Sherburn Hill meant for the first time our family could move out from the council house and into our own home. This was just up the hill in East Stanley. Having said all that, I only have fond memories of South Stanley and I wouldn't change a thing about my early years there.

Towards the end of my final year at school I was losing interest in my academic studies. Although the country was suffering an economic depression, the education we received at Tanfield was excellent. I'd been fortunate enough to pass the Eleven-plus exam to get into a grammar, but I was throwing away my education by being only interested in football. I had dreams of playing for England, so why should I bother with my English and maths O-Levels? I'm sure thousands of boys before and after me have had the same thought process and it's something professional clubs have tried to tackle after the 1970s. I do remember my mother stressing the importance of educational achievement, 'just in case', but of course I dismissed that advice.

We had a very strict headmaster at school called Dr Sharp. He was legendary. Any disobedience and the cane came out: hand or arse, he didn't seem to mind. There were about 800 kids at the school and lunchtime (we called it dinner) was a noisy affair, but when the Doc entered the hall, those assembled fell silent. The whole room avoided eye contact with him. One day, not too far off from the O-Level exams, I was summoned to his office. On the way I wondered which offence I'd been observed committing and had a couple of ideas, but when I went in he told me there were concerns that I was neglecting my studies because of football. He told me that if I failed my exams he would ban me from signing for Arsenal as an apprentice. Looking back, I'm sure he wouldn't have been able to do that, but I'll always be grateful for that threat because it ensured I worked hard at school for my final exams. Little did I know then how important that would be. I must give a mention to one of my teachers from the primary school, Greenland, called Miss Handy. She would always have a quiet word with me and tell me that I would always do well in my studies if I believed in myself. It was her sensitive encouragement just as much as the Doc's methods that worked.

I finished school in the summer of 1975, fortunately with good O-Levels. I signed my apprentice forms for Arsenal on 21 August, for a two-year period. I had the summer months at home then moved to London for the start of the 1975/76 season. No matter how hard a club tries to prepare and support a 16-year-old child moving away from home, it's not easy. Once it finally dawned on me that I wasn't heading home on the train every Sunday evening I became very homesick. I'd left a loving home in a very tight-knit mining community to live in digs in the capital city of England.

North London in the 1970s was a far cry from home. I lived in digs with another apprentice from Mansfield called Carl. We lived on Arnos Grove in Southgate. His homesickness was worse than mine: I woke one morning to find a note from him on my bed telling me he could bear it no longer and he was going home immediately.

I must admit, I was close to following him to King's Cross and jumping on the first train heading north too. One thing that helped me was receiving letters from home. I still have a shoebox full of them, many of which were from my good school friends, Graham Kirtley, Gordon Baker and Eric Tregonning. Graham and Gordon are supporters who have followed Newcastle United their whole life and still have season tickets. Treg was a Sunderland supporter with great football skills. Unlike me, he made the decision early regarding his future and passed up any trials to concentrate on his studies. He became a dentist and practised in Stanley his whole career.

Once again, the club did what they could to help with my homesickness. I was a bit young to go to pubs, but I do remember going on my own to the pictures in Leicester Square and being amazed by the volume of people milling about the place. My time in Southgate came to an end one evening when the train bringing me back from Newcastle got into King's Cross late, and when I got to the digs the landlady refused to let me in. I had to find a telephone box to call home. In a panic, my mam contacted a distant relative, who happened to be a retired police inspector down in Islington. He drove across London to get me. I ended up staying with Uncle Jim and Aunty Margaret for about six months. I couldn't impose myself on them for ever, so the club arranged for me to move in with the family of one of the other boys in the team, Colin Brooks. They lived in Worcester Park near Guildford in Surrey. This was much more like being back in a family atmosphere, I'm sure something that also gave my parents a lot of relief. I remember going down to Box Hill and enjoying the Surrey North Downs. Colin was released and started working for his dad's roofing business, and Arsenal decided I should move again. This time they put me in digs in Barnet, north London. I would get picked up every day in Cockfosters to take me to the training ground.

On the football pitch things were going well. I continued playing in the South East Counties League, then progressed to the reserves, playing in the Football Combination. I've kept a photo of a couple of us apprentices standing with Malcolm Macdonald, one of my Newcastle heroes, who was then an Arsenal player. Many of my team-mates eventually went on to become household names; I played alongside fellow young hopefuls such as David O'Leary, Frank Stapleton, Graham Rix and Wilf Rostron. Older players such as John Radford and big Terry Mancini sometimes played in the reserves.

It was around this time that I started taking an interest in the work of the physiotherapist, Fred Street. Bertie Mee had encouraged Fred to train as a physio several years earlier, and then when the opportunity came up he had him transferred to Arsenal. Bertie also had an interest in injuries and rehabilitation. I would observe what Fred did and said to the players when he was treating them. He'd also become England physio shortly before I joined the club, so he had everyone's respect.

The turning point for my career as a footballer was probably an incident I had as a spectator that happened after the Spurs versus Newcastle League Cup semi-final first leg at White Hart Lane on the evening of 14 January 1976. I'd been an apprentice for about six months and, despite missing home desperately, I was successful on the pitch. The semi-final was an opportunity to meet some of my mates from Stanley who had travelled down for the match. There was nothing better than a bit of the North East coming into my London life, even if it was for a matter of hours. The match itself ended in a 1-0 victory for Spurs but there was still a lot of hope for the return fixture a week later. I said goodbye to my Stanley friend, Stephen McPhail, and headed towards the Seven Sisters Tube station, dealing with the lump in my throat. As I left Stephen, I carefully hid my scarf in my trousers pocket; after all, football hooliganism was a significant problem at that time.

I must have been spotted wearing the scarf before I hid it; I heard a shout and turned to see a gang of 10 to 15 Spurs supporters running towards me. They were coming at me so quickly, I barely had time to kick the first one in the midriff and land a punch on a second attacker before I was submerged in a melee of fists and feet. I tried to retaliate but quickly decided the only option was to curl up. I took a lot of kicks to the head and chest. At some point I lost consciousness. When I woke up I was lying in a garden minus my coat, with my shirt ripped. My scarf was gone, too. Once I'd gathered my thoughts, I hobbled to the Tube station and got myself back to Worcester Park train station in Surrey. What the people on the Tube thought about a bloodied and bruised 17-year-old boy in a shredded shirt sitting beside them, I'll never know because they never asked. I'm certain, had I been in Newcastle, a mother hen would have helped me. At the time I was just thankful that I manged to get away relatively unscathed, although my chest and head hurt a lot.

I'd taken several heavy blows to my face and head in fights before this, but I'd never been knocked unconscious. The following day I felt shocking; I had headaches, felt sick and was generally out of sorts. I had what the doctors today would call post-concussion syndrome, a constellation of symptoms that can occur after a moderate head injury. The club decided I would be better off at home, so I headed north for three weeks. I remember Alan Oliver the famous sports reporter wrote a piece on the assault for the *Evening Chronicle*. After returning to training and playing I struggled with pain in my chest for another four weeks, probably due to cracked ribs. After that it was a struggle to regain full fitness.

Shortly after that event, in March, we had the opportunity to watch a midweek match between Newcastle and Arsenal. A group of us apprentices were sat behind the Arsenal team bench. I was beside David O'Leary. I must have still been indignant following my assault, so I wore a black-and-white hat and got a right bollocking for it at training the next day. Things weren't helped when Bertie Mee resigned at the end of the 1975/76 season. His replacement was Terry Neill, who travelled the short distance from Spurs. I started the following season well enough, but then suffered a bad ankle injury that kept me out for a further six weeks. And then came the discussion no aspiring footballer wants. The new manager Neill had taken a look at me and decided I would never be in the club's plans. I was part of a mass clear-out that he was having. This came quite early into the new season, while I was still recovering from the ankle sprain. But that was that … I was out. Close to my 18th birthday, heading home with my dreams in tatters. Bizarrely, the best way I had of dealing with it was repeating the mantra that I just wasn't good enough. Perhaps I knew in my heart of hearts that I *wasn't* good enough.

Chapter 2

Fulham

MY PRIORITY on returning home was getting another chance at another club. My ankle wasn't healing I as would like, but I was desperate. The manager of York City, Wilf McGuiness, was keen to give me a trial. When he took over at York in 1975 they were a Second Division club but had struggled after Wilf arrived. By October 1976 they were sinking. Unfortunately, I was of no help and I did myself no favours. I was unfit and injured when I played for the reserve team midweek against Grimsby Town on 12 October. After a particularly sorry performance that was the end to my football career. It taught me a lesson for my future as a physio, that it just isn't worth playing while unfit and injured. It took several weeks and a visit to an orthopaedic specialist with stress X-rays to eventually learn that I'd completely ruptured my lateral ligament complex. My joint was, in effect, unstable. I was eventually able to rehab it back to a good function for football but, as I'd already concluded, it didn't avoid the fact that I was never going to be good enough to play professionally.

I needed to decide what my future was. I was interested in physiotherapy, so I spoke to Fred Street about it. He recommended that I study remedial gymnastics, a form of rehabilitation based predominantly on exercise therapy. Its origins came from the

Second World War, successfully combining exercise and physical therapy for injured soldiers. The thought had occasionally crossed my mind while I was at school that a career in medicine would be very rewarding and interesting. I believed that I was already too late to go down that route, but I hoped I was able to get a place on the remedial gymnastics course, not particularly to get back into football, but because musculoskeletal pathology and treatment interested me.

The course was based at Pinderfields Hospital in Wakefield. I contacted the course lead, Paddy Armour, with the help of Fred. He told me the earliest entry date I could get would be September 1977, plus I would need at least an A-Level in biology. So, I enrolled for that at night class and looked for work in the meantime. I took a job cleaning the streets with a tractor. My first day was in Byker. The farmer had given me a list of streets to do. It was impossible to complete without working an extra three to four hours without a break. To make matters worse, on the way back the tractor went over a bump going down Bensham bank, causing the driver's side window to fall in and smash into tiny cubes of glass all over me and the cab. When I finally got back to the depot the farmer gave me £4 for the day's work and whinged about his window; I packed my job in there and then.

I was lucky enough to get a labouring job in my dad's blossoming engineering company in Sherburn Hill. The interviews for Pinderfields came and went. I know of no other job interview where you also had to literally do cartwheels, but that's one of the things I had to do. Just as well I practised for it! If anyone is interested in becoming a remedial gymnast, that won't be possible as the profession merged with the physiotherapy profession in November 1985.

As things worked out, Paddy later said the A-Level was not necessary, so I confirmed my place in Pinderfields starting in the late summer of 1977. The female students were resident in the nursing home, while all the males were housed in an old vicarage. The course was hard work but we had plenty of time to socialise. It was a brilliant time. I remember after classes somebody would make a big brew of tea for all of us, a packet of digestives was passed around and we then would usually do a couple of hours work before hitting Wakefield or Pontefract for beers. Leeds was just up the road as well. We also had regular parties in the vicarage. I have a memory of one where someone was riding a moped up and down the stairs in the vicarage. I'd never seen the guy before. I suppose the drink-driving laws don't apply to staircases. I developed friendships that I've maintained to this day. Dave Lowe emigrated to Canada, as did Nick Elbrow. Neil Metcalfe stayed in England and became a football physio as well.

Paddy Armour, the college principal, had recently established the medical department of the FA at that time. He started up the framework of the FA's approach to injuries and medical issues. This training has now become very complex and involves intensive courses on medical emergencies and resuscitation for the club physiotherapists and doctors. Paddy was old-school, always wore an immaculate white coat and came across like a stern sergeant major during lectures and practicals, but he was very knowledgeable in body mechanics, or kinesiology as it's called today. He retired and was replaced by Alan Hodgson, who later became employed by the FA and became Director of the FA's Medical Department for many years. So, remedial gymnasts were instrumental in creating the FA's medical infrastructure.

By the time I started my course in Wakefield my ankle had healed and was sufficiently stable for me to play some matches for Durham City in the Northern League during 1977/78. When I started the final year of my course I went on placement to

Northumberland. I also changed football clubs to Cramlington New Town in the Northern Alliance. I scored all four goals in my winning debut against local rivals Morpeth Town.

For my student placement I did six months in Ashington General Hospital and six months in Hartford Hall near Bedlington. If I learned one thing from my time in Ashington General, it was that I wasn't suited to NHS work. I remember working on the maternity ward, where the physiotherapists gave post-natal care to the mothers. I was allowed to observe a birth. When the mother was asked for permission, she said, 'Ah divvent care who's watchin', just get it oot!' I was told to stand down at the 'business end', behind the midwives. Everything seemed to be going fine; the baby's head popped out, but the midwives were concerned about the baby's cord around its neck. The team was very professional as it went into action, but the mild panic mixed with scenes of blood and slime and the little baby's blue face brought me out in an intense sweat. Feeling dizzy and thirsty, I thought I was going to faint. I searched out a wall that I could slide myself down discreetly, but happily they rapidly delivered the baby and I regained my composure, narrowly avoiding passing out on the delivery room floor.

Hartford Hall was more my place. It was a rehabilitation centre for injured Northumberland miners, funded by the National Union of Miners with the care delivered by the NHS. When I started it was purely for miners. The men there were resident while having their treatment. They had a variety of injuries ranging from trauma due to unfortunate encounters with mining machinery, to knee and back problems from constant bending and twisting.

Remedial gymnastics and physiotherapy were still separate professions at the time. There were three physios, Joyce, Joan and Heather, and one remedial gymnast. The remedial gymnast was Jimmy Luke, ex-army who garnered the miners' respect through his communication skills and attention to detail. Not to be outdone, the female therapists gave as good as they got from their tough Northumbrian clients! Not long after I started, we were given a tour of Ellington Colliery. At the time it was one of the largest deep mines in the world. Although relatively modern in terms of the previous 200 years of mining, it was still a real eye-opener and retained some of the older practices. For example, they still used pit ponies.

The cage experience down was fine, in a well-lit roomy automated elevator. The scene outside the shaft exit looked and sounded like the inside of a factory or warehouse. The men told me their enemy was methane gas, or firedamp. This was invisible but very flammable; once ignited, the methane causes the coal dust in the atmosphere to explode so the pit had to be well ventilated. They used large electric fans for this, but many years ago they had to fire up huge coal furnaces below the ground to circulate the air (the hot gases went up a shaft, pulling fresh air down another shaft into the pit).

We had electric lights to illuminate the space and we got into a small train that took us for about three miles. After that they took us to an old section of the mine; we had to crawl on to a coal conveyor belt and lie on it. That took us a further two miles. Once we got off that, the rest of the way was on foot. On this line the coalface was six miles out below the North Sea, but some lines went for 15 miles. I tried not to imagine the tons of rock and water above our heads. As we went in, the roof got lower and lower, with occasional horizontal girders to bang your head on. The miners seemed to prefer to walk in a squat position, on their 'hunkers', but I ended up stooping forwards then went on my hands and knees at one point after I'd banged my head on the roof two or three times. The problem with that method is that there are jagged bits of stone on the hard, rock floor so the knees can take very little of that until you have to go back to the 'squat walk'.

Next they took us to some modern workings. It was a privilege to get to the coalface where the men had put up the hydraulic pit props and were extracting the coal with cutting machines and electric picks. Despite the ventilation it was incredibly hot and pitch black, so we needed the use of the electric torches on our helmets to see where we were going. What a racket the machines made, throwing up coal dust while they were cutting out the coal. It takes a certain type of person to do this job well. A lot of the time the men still worked in that crouched position, while breathing in clouds of black dust, despite their masks. It's a job that requires physical fitness, no doubt about it. I could see why a dedicated rehab centre was useful.

Back at Hartford Hall they'd constructed an obstacle course that resembled the underground conditions, low roof, twists and turns. It was a very effective way of assessing the men's progress. Meniscal injuries were common, so the 'squat walk' was often difficult for their knees. In the remedial gymnastics style we had a training hall where you stood on a table in the middle and barked out instructions to the men like an army PT instructor. But it seemed to work, and the men put in a lot of effort. We would then break out to smaller group therapy for specific injuries. Once or twice a year the Northumberland miners would compete in sports against the Durham miners, who were based at the Hermitage in Chester-le-Street. These were usually *very* competitive events.

One of the stranger things that happened was that the miners had a trip out every Thursday night. They were given free beer tokens and we took them up to Bedlington Top Club in a minibus where the men got 'smashed' (we did too, if we weren't on duty).

There were always a few hangovers for the following day's morning session. On a Friday afternoon they took it easy and played games such as bowls and quoits. This was the era of the first Thatcher government and at that time men were still optimistic about the UK mining industry. Obviously, the situation deteriorated rapidly after that and the rehab centre has closed now, as there are no more pits. I have no doubt someone behind a desk would have eventually put a stop to the sessions on free beer tokens. Suffice it to say, we all loved the Bedlington nights out.

I must mention one of the classic stories, but it did happen. A visiting hand surgeon was assessing a muckle miner's huge hands and fat fingers after he'd crushed a hand inside a piece of machinery. The surgeon was most impressed with his own surgical skills, when the miner asked, while examining in his own hands intently, 'So, will I be able to play the piano?' He made 'piano-playing' movements with his fingers. The surgeon inspected his hands once more and gave a positive prognosis: 'Yes, of course. I don't see why not,' to which the miner replied, 'That's great, doc, 'cos I couldn't play beforehand.' The look on the surgeon's face was priceless!

I was awarded my certificate from the College of Remedial Gymnastics and Recreational Therapy, Pinderfields General Hospital Wakefield on Wednesday, 30 April 1980 (I obtained a further Chartered Physiotherapist qualification later). From the contacts I made in Northumberland, the first job I did after qualifying was in Northgate Hospital near Morpeth. This involved working with physically and mentally handicapped children. I continued playing football at that time, still turning out for Cramlington New Town. I also managed to take part in the first-ever Great North Run in June, with no distance training whatsoever. My lowly position reflected that!

It was while working in Morpeth that I had the greatest break I could have in football. Malcolm Macdonald was the Fulham FC manager, and his physio, John Clinkard, was leaving for Everton. In a passing conversation, Malcolm asked Fred Street if he knew of any suitable replacements. Fred immediately thought of me. I'll always be grateful to Fred for his recommendation to Supermac. Malcolm phoned me and asked if I could make it to London for the following morning, which was a Saturday. Fulham were at home and had a three o'clock later that day. I told him of course I would be there, but when I came to look for trains or flights, nothing worked. Late in the evening I decided to get some sleep and drive down, so I set off from Newcastle at 3.30am, arriving at Craven Cottage for 9.30am. Immediately after the interview, Malcolm told me I had the job. He'd been particularly impressed by my decision to drive through the night to get there.

So, that was it, I worked my notice in the NHS and started as a football physiotherapist in October 1981 at the age of 23. I was the youngest in the Football League at that time. It sounds old-fashioned now but the club put an advert in the programme seeking temporary accommodation for me for two weeks while I looked for a place to live. Alan and Vanessa Fisher lived right beside the ground and they answered the call to put me up for two weeks, which ended up being two years! I became part of their family.

When I worked at my first match in November 1981, Fulham were in the Third Division. However, in less than a year Malcolm had transformed the team, as a young manager. Without bringing in new players he'd developed the team to one that played with a lot of style, their method fast and direct, while retaining possession. As a manager and as a person Malcolm was very good to me. He was quietly spoken and considered, but always supportive. To me he came across as very intelligent and articulate. Put it this way, he would usually sit doing the *Times* crossword and complete it, when I had no idea what half of the clues meant. A lot of thought went into his football decision-making, and he was usually correct.

I always remember my first Christmas there, recently arrived and knowing very few people in London; Malcolm invited me to his house in Bedfordshire to spend Christmas with his wife and girls. I think that gives you a measure of the man. That aside, he was one of the best managers I worked under. His man-management skills were second to none. I previously mentioned the photograph with Supermac in his Arsenal days talking to some of the apprentices, and I'm one of them. He always said he remembered me from then, even if he didn't really!

My old reserves team-mate from Arsenal, Terry Mancini, was there as a coach, working alongside assistant manager Ray Harford. Another ex-Arsenal regular there on the coaching staff was George Armstrong. I never crossed paths with Geordie while I was at Arsenal, but he became firm friends at Fulham. It was the North East connection that helped establish the bond. Ray Harford also became a good friend. Malcolm would be the first to admit that Ray was an important factor in winning promotion to the Second Division at the end of the 1981/82 season (Kenny Dalglish similarly lauded Ray years later when Blackburn won the Premier League with Ray as the first-team coach).

It was Roger Brown's header against Lincoln City on the last day of the season that clinched the third and final promotion spot for us. Lincoln were in fourth place so the 1-1 draw at Craven Cottage saw us through. Other notable players of that era were Tony Gale, Gordon Davies, Ray Lewington, Dean Coney, Paul Parker and Gerry Peyton. I became friendly and socialised with Ray Lewington and Tony Gale, both of whom were the same age as me. I became godfather to Ray's son, Craig. In fact, Ray still sends my parents a Christmas card every year. The last time he saw me, down at Crystal Palace, he introduced me to Roy Hodgson and reminded me of a story that he also told to Roy: I played for Ray's Sunday team. We played all over London. Once we were playing away somewhere in the East End and some cockney lad had been winding me up most of the match, so we had a bit of a barney. No doubt he was a Millwall supporter. He started coming out with the 'I'm an Eastender gangster' bollocks. He then told me he was going to get his shotgun out of the car, come back and blast me with it. Of course, that made no difference to me; I told him to go and get it. Ray assured me later that he *was* from a gangster family and there was a fair chance that he did have a gun in his car! Anyway, as Ray told Roy, I didn't back down. Never back down.

Ray Houghton was signed for the following season, and we started promisingly. A red-letter day for me was the day we visited Newcastle at St James'. The stadium was full and the Toon supporters were on form. There's a great photo in the book of Supermac, Ray Harford and me squeezing ourselves into the dugout. There were no 20-seat all-weather dugouts with heated seats in those days, just a concrete or brick square structure with a wooden bench cemented in. The Geordies gave Supermac a tremendous welcome despite anticipating putting one over on their hero. That wasn't to be: Fulham were on fire that day, playing in a style similar to that of the entertainers that were yet to grace the ground. The whole stadium was shocked when Malcolm's team scored three quick goals, making it look effortless. Even Kevin Keegan playing in the Newcastle team wasn't enough to get them back into the match, eventually losing 4-1.

As the second half ticked down, the Newcastle supporters realised they were beaten. I was astonished to see them begin to applaud the Fulham players when they impressed with an attack or attempt on goal. At the final whistle they gave the Fulham players a standing ovation as they left the pitch. I've never seen that happen anywhere since. A cynic might say they were just hoping Malcolm would come back as manager. They probably were, but that day they were simply showing their appreciation of a wonderful display. Experiencing that atmosphere, I knew then that St James' Park was where I belonged. Ray Lewington stayed up with me after the match. I took him to Parker's nightclub in Stanley. That was a bit of an eye-opener to someone from West London! A few years later Barry Venison told me he'd taken Ally McCoist to the other Stanley nightclub, the 'Hunt'.

Despite the demolition of Newcastle that day, we didn't gain promotion. A mostly forgotten series of events contributed to us failing to go up. We were looking good for the run-in, but we lost four of our last five matches. Before that run, we had a five-point advantage. By the final fixture we'd thrown that away. On the last day, Leicester, who were playing at home, only had to beat Burnley, who were struggling near the bottom of the league. We were away to Derby and we needed to win, but so did Derby because they were battling relegation. As it turned out, Leicester drew with Burnley, so we could have been promoted. At the Baseball Ground, Derby scored to take the lead in the 71st minute. When they scored, the Derby fans invaded the pitch. It took a while for the police to clear them off, but more and more fans spilled off the terraces and encroached on the playing surface. One fan even kicked Robert Wilson when he was running down the wing. Where we were in the dugout, the police formed a protective cordon around us, making it difficult to see the match. There was real hostility there, but we were focused on the excitement and despair of the last 15 to 20 desperate minutes; trying to ignore the simmering threat around us. Ray Harford and I had to stand away from the dugout to see the play, but the police weren't happy with that.

The referee blew his whistle in the 89th minute. It later transpired that this was for offside, and he still had 78 seconds left to go. The crowd invaded the pitch once more and a lot of them started aggressively milling around us. We were ushered down the tunnel, and the players started arriving at intervals. Most of the players said they'd been physically assaulted. Jeff Hopkins came in with his shirt in tatters and smashed a cup off the wall. Many of the other players had had their shirts ripped off their backs. The referee decided it was too unsafe to complete the match, so he abandoned it. As always, I was the last to leave the dressing room. Just before I left with the kitman and coach driver, the referee came in and admitted to me that he would have abandoned the match earlier if the Fulham players hadn't been so well behaved throughout. If any of them, the staff or Malcolm, had complained any more about the encroachment and provocation earlier, he would have abandoned it earlier.

Malcolm was understandably annoyed; he immediately protested and appealed for the match to be replayed. He found unexpected allies in the Derby chairman Mike Watterson and the Leicester manager Gordon Milne. The Football League secretary, Graham Kelly, didn't see it that way. He refused to replay the match despite a second appeal. It was a terrible way to end such a promising season. Malcolm took it hard, and things were never the same. The following season we struggled; Malcolm resigned in April amid frenzied press interest in his domestic situation. This left Ray Harford in charge for the rest of the season.

Did I mention that I played for Fulham Reserves? Well, yes I did, in the Football Combination. I played mainly in the 1983/84 season, some eight years after playing for Arsenal in the same league. Terry Mancini was the reserves' player-manager. So, despite being the physio, I also played: centre-forward. I only had one request and that was that the coach driver would bring my 'bucket and sponge' on if a player was injured. This was still the days of the magic sponge. Poor guy was a bit dyspraxic. He would run on with such enthusiasm but poor coordination, so by the time he arrived the bucket was empty and most of its contents were all over him. I reverted to getting my own magic sponge.

Several weeks after playing a reserve match I was reminded of it by Terry Mancini. We'd played Watford Reserves at Vicarage Road. Terry confessed to me that the Orient manager, Frank Clark, had been watching one of the matches. He approached Terry afterwards and asked about the availability of the centre-forward, Derek Wright, only to be told, 'Fuck off, you're not having my physiotherapist!' Many years later Frank confirmed this a couple of times when I bumped into him in Newcastle. If only, I might have been a star centre-forward for Leyton Orient FC.

My second fortunate break in football physio came shortly after the start of 1984/85. Newcastle had just been promoted to the First Division, but Arthur Cox and Kevin Keegan had left before the start of the season. Jack Charlton had taken over. He needed a physiotherapist, after the current one, Ian Liversedge, announced that he was leaving to go to Oldham. The club doctor, Keith Beveridge, was on the lookout. One of the physios I worked with at Northumberland Health Authority, Cath Anderson, recommended me to her brother, Peter Anderson, who was the assistant doctor at the club. One thing led to another and Dr Beveridge contacted me. Newcastle's next match was in London against QPR in the league, so I went to the hotel to meet Jack and the doc after they had dinner. I met for the interview on 21 September 1984. I remember the date because it was the night before the famous 5-5 draw against Rangers on the plastic pitch at Loftus Road. A brief chat with a fellow Geordie, mainly about fishing, which I know nothing about, and a bit about my background in football, and I was offered the job! Jack and the doc took me straight down the stairs and introduced me to some of the lads. I was on my way back to Newcastle and couldn't wait to get started. Ray Harford was very understanding; he knew of my ties to the North East and understood why I wanted to return to Newcastle.

Chapter 3

Newcastle

BEFORE THE start of the 1982/83 season, Newcastle were in the Second Division and at a low ebb. With what little money he was given, manager Arthur Cox had pulled off a masterstroke and brought Kevin Keegan to the club. It took a couple of years, but by the end of 1983/84 Arthur's team had secured promotion. The club was emerging from one of its darkest periods; the fans were still buoyed by the 'Keegan effect', even though their hero had gone, along with Terry Mac. To be fair, the chairman, Stan Seymour, had worked hard to improve the club's finances, but this meant Arthur still had very little money to spend on players. This was one of the reasons he left after securing promotion. His replacement was Jack Charlton.

Before I arrived, the season had started well, Big Jack's team winning the first three matches. We then lost three and had a few draws. My first match as NUFC physiotherapist was away to Ipswich, Tuesday, 30 October 1984. This was also my first day in the job. I was very apprehensive going into that match; I felt unprepared as I'd only just managed to get up from London. I still remember that day clearly and will never forget how kind Peter Beardsley, Kenny Wharton and captain Glenn Roeder were to me. They went out of their way to greet me and then introduce me to the rest of the team. They were brilliant and I'll always appreciate that kindness. It was the League Cup third round, first leg. We drew 1-1. There were some great players in that team as well as Kenny, Peter and Glen. Chris Waddle was up front, Dave McCreery in midfield, Wes Sanders centre-half and, of course, the great Toon servant, John Anderson. My next match was the following Saturday, away against Luton; that finished as yet another draw. Then came the replay against Ipswich. I was so thrilled to sit on the home bench with the excited supporters willing the Toon into the next round. Alas, it wasn't to be, and we lost 2-1.

My first home fixture in the league was Saturday, 10 November when we beat Chelsea 2-1. That was a great experience: raucous crowd, great joy from the stands and the pleasure of a win. The following Sunday we went down 2-0 at home to Liverpool. After that, it didn't take long for the magnitude of the club's situation to become apparent to me. There was already a lot of pressure on Jack from the press and fans. As the season progressed and the team slipped down the table, Jack brought in Pat Heard, George Reilly and Tony Cunningham. George and Tony were big lads for the rest of the team to target. Many fans disliked the long-ball game and some openly criticised the manager for it, especially when Chris Waddle and Peter Beardsley were put out on the wings. But the lads gained enough points to finish 14th. Jack always gave as good as he got in the papers and said the club's debt had to be acknowledged as a reason why there hadn't been bigger signings and why the team played in the style he directed.

The training ground at Benwell reflected the club's situation: the facilities were terrible, tiny changing rooms and treatment rooms, reminiscent of a scout hut condemned by wet rot. The walls that weren't wooden were unpainted breeze block, and a sorry-looking rusty multigym sat neglected in the corner. The place had a permanent smell of damp and mould. The playing area was passable, probably big enough for four full-size pitches, but surrounded by houses. The facilities were not good enough for a club the size of Newcastle. This was a First Division club with Fourth Division facilities. I'd just come from Fulham, in the division below. They trained at the Bank of England Sports Centre in Roehampton: endless manicured pitches, grass tennis courts, gym, sports hall, swimming pool and lavish clubhouse.

I've always been obsessively tidy so I set about improving the treatment facilities as best as I could. I enrolled some of the young lads to give the place a spruce up while I scrubbed the rust off the multigym with a metal brush, then oiled it down. The first boy I collared was Paul Gascoigne. The coach, Colin Suggett, had started calling him Gazza. In hindsight, he probably wasn't my best choice for a cleaner. Gazza's problem was he wouldn't shut up. The lad was always manic, up to something or wanting to chatter away. He was 17 at the time and, despite me only being 26, he insisted on calling me Mr Wright. He would get his broom, while sweeping up and chatting away to me, then place his palms on the end of the handle and rest his chin on his hands while telling me some bollocks about nefarious happenings in Dunston or something his sister had told him five weeks earlier. He must have thought this broom position gave him some sort of free pass to stop work. I had to ban him from talking while sweeping up.

Another time I was in a hurry to lock up. I'd sent Gazza into the treatment room to tidy up. It was for the final Friday afternoon inspection I'd instituted. It had gone suspiciously quiet, so I went in to see what he was doing. He was nowhere to be seen, which was impossible as there was only one door. I was looking up at the ceiling to see if he'd crawled up into the roof space. Out of the corner of my eye, something moved in the big industrial dryer we had for the players' kit. Gazza had climbed in and locked himself inside, sitting with his face plastered against the glass and tongue hanging out, trying to look like a dead Quasimodo. He could be a proper handful, but Colin was great at keeping a lid on his antics, having been his youth-team coach alongside Jimmy Nelson when they won the FA Trophy.

Two lads who I would be work colleagues alongside later in my career were Paul Ferris, from Lisburn in Northern Ireland, and Cruddas Park's own John Carver. Both were injured, along with Peter Haddock, who was in a plaster cast for a medial ligament rupture. Paul, nicknamed Ferra, and JC were my first injuries. JC was plagued by a recurrent quadriceps tear that wouldn't heal, eventually requiring surgery. Ferra was only a kid, but he was a full professional; he spent a long time in my treatment room. He was bright as a button, a thinker. We talked a lot about current affairs. Irish politics was important to him because it had directly affected his family: Catholics in a predominantly Protestant town. I confess my knowledge of Irish history and politics wasn't great. He said I was a classic 'John Bull'. I had to look that up but had to agree that his assessment was fairly accurate.

I suspected JC and Ferra's lifestyle wasn't helping their injuries, so I threatened to visit their rented flat in Jesmond. Somehow Paul's claim that every meal was home-cooked 'meat and two veg' didn't ring true. I knew they thought I wouldn't go, so one weekday evening I paid them a surprise visit. The inspection didn't start too well. The hallway was lit in a dull crimson by a bare 25-watt lightbulb, giving the impression of an entrance to a seedy brothel. The sitting room wasn't any better, resembling a hovel. Plates were strewn about the floor and empty cans of 'full-fat' pop and Red Stripe nestled among chocolate bar wrappers on the kitchen table. Sure enough, the fridge was almost empty other than half a dozen beer bottles, some cheese, a couple of sprouting potatoes and more bars of chocolate. Curly Wurly seemed to be their favourite. We all had a good laugh about it because they couldn't believe I would catch them out. I did point out that their lifestyle wasn't the best for professional athletes. It was a real shame, but John wasn't long at the club after that and was released to go to play for Cardiff.

On the pitch the team was perceived to have struggled in Jack's first season, but he'd managed to keep them in the top flight, even though we'd drifted down the table as the season went on. For the new campaign he had players to call on such as Chris Waddle and Peter Beardsley, not to mention Gazza on the fringes. There were also seasoned professionals such as Jeff Clarke, John Anderson and Dave McCreery. There was a lot to look forward to.

As soon as the season ended, we left for a post-season tour of New Zealand. Jack didn't travel so Willie McFaul the first-team coach was in charge. The lads weren't too pleased in having to travel halfway around the world when what they really wanted to do was take a well-earned break from football to recharge the batteries for another season. The week before we left, I broke my fifth metatarsal playing for Chris Waddle's Sunday League team, Gateshead Azure Blue. The orthopod wanted to put my foot in a plaster cast, but I wouldn't have that because it meant I wouldn't have been able to travel.

We played four matches in New Zealand against the national team, then two in Fiji against their national team. I must say the two countries were very beautiful in very different ways. In New Zealand we played in Christchurch, Wellington, Auckland and Napier. Somewhere on the North Island, Gazza treated himself to getting his hair dyed, so for the rest of the trip he was the proud owner of bleached blond curls. The fixtures came thick and fast, so the lads did no training, just played. Despite my broken foot I got on the subs' bench for the final match against Fiji but never came on, other than as physio. Towards the end, George Reilly went down right at the far corner of the pitch, howling in agony. I had to sprint on, with my broken foot killing me every time it hit the ground, only for George to jump up as soon as I got there with all the lads having a good laugh at my expense.

The first leg of the return flights was Fiji to Los Angeles, and it's without doubt the worst flight I, and probably most of the other guys, have ever had. Unbeknown to us, the pilot was trying to navigate around a storm at the time; the Jumbo we were on suddenly dropped what felt like about 500 feet then made a loud bang before dropping another 300 feet with an even louder bang. Trolleys were flung about. Anyone not fastened in became weightless, some even hit their heads on the roof and had minor head injuries. Air stewardesses were in tears. You know something's not right when *they're* crying. Honestly, I thought the second bang was us crashing. I happened to be sitting beside Gazza, who was immediately hysterical. He was in floods of tears and convinced himself we were all going to die. I was just relieved we *hadn't* died, but for the rest of the flight the lad was in bits. Something my mother has always remembered, when we finally arrived back at Newcastle airport, she was there to give me a lift home. I gave her a hug, then Gazza came up and gave her a big hug as well. In the car he proceeded to tell my parents how we all nearly died in the skies over the Pacific. In his autobiography, *Gazza: My Story*, he says that he was 'shit-scared' during his first-ever flight to Toulon in 1987 with England Under-21s. He must have totally banished the memory of the LA flight from his memory!

We weren't long back from the trip when I went to the Bruce Springsteen concert at St James' and met a girl called Lisa who became my girlfriend and was to become my wife and the mother of my eldest son, Jonathan. That summer was a good time, back home among my people, hanging out with my old mates from school.

The prospect of a full season coming up with the Toon was also exciting. By the time pre-season training came around, Gazza had long forgotten the flight from hell, and his brown hair coming through at the roots was betraying his bleached 80s bouffant. I was preparing to go home for the day when he came running into the treatment room at Benwell. 'Mr Wright, Mr Wright, Ave forgot me bus fare,' he said.

'What?'

'Ave forgot me bus fare, man!' I thought he was cadging some money, which was fair enough.

'Here, I'll give you some, is 20 pence enough?'

'Eh? Nor, nor, nor; A divvent want yer money, Mr Wright. Am gannin' carol singin' fer it.'

'It's July, ye daft bugger.'

'Aye, doesn't matter. Just watch.' He ran off down the hill towards Gibside Gardens. Every ten yards or so he looked back to make sure I was still watching, waving each time. He started at the first door and worked his way down the hill. He started with 'Hark, the Herald Angels Sing', did that a couple of times then went on to 'We Wish You a Merry Christmas'. Each time he came back down the path he gave the gladiatorial thumbs-down, but he emerged from the fourth garden triumphant and gave the thumbs-up. He sprinted back up the hill.

'There ye gan, Mr Wright. A telt ye!' He proudly displayed his rewards then set off for the bus back to Dunston. 'See ye the morra, Mr Wright.'

* * *

We were at St James' for a pre-season friendly against Sheffield United. There were fewer than 10,000 in the ground. The team weren't on best form; it didn't help that Chris Waddle had been sold to Spurs. A significant section of the supporters in the Gallowgate jeered and barracked Jack throughout the game, calling for him to go. That was enough abuse for the big man. I remember him muttering something about some of the support at the time we were sat in the dugout. I never supposed a small group of disgruntled lads in a half-empty stadium was enough to tip him over the edge, but it was. To be fair to Jack, my recollection is that the fans giving him a hard time had kept up the harassment for the whole match. Ray Lewington was playing for Sheffield at that time and was heading back to London by train. I was going to give him a lift to Central Station and was waiting out in the foyer of the old stand when Jack walked by, still muttering.

'That's it, Derek, I've fuckin' had enough of this,' he said as he passed me. Ray came out, I took him to the station, dropped him off and put the radio on. The news was already reporting that he'd gone. Jack had resigned! He'll always be a North East hero. He went on to become an Irish hero after that.

Willie McFaul was installed as caretaker manager. I'd established a good working relationship with Willie, so the transition for me was smooth; he'd been at the Toon for years. He was a great guy, very good with the players and a good coach. He knew his football. The season started well for the team and Willie was given a permanent deal. Ferra managed to seriously damage his knee right at the start of Willie's tenure. From the mechanism, I thought he might have done his anterior cruciate ligament (ACL).

To be more specific, I thought at the time that Ferra had ruptured his medial collateral ligament (MCL) and *possibly* his ACL. Twenty minutes later, his knee had filled with blood, making an ACL injury more likely in my mind. I took Paul to the surgeon's offices in Jesmond later that day. His diagnosis was more favourable than mine: MCL partial tear. A rupture is a complete tear. Although the MCL is very important to the knee's stability, even a complete rupture is likely to heal over time. However, a complete rupture of the ACL is crucial in creating instability in the knee and rarely heals without surgery to correct that instability. Until not too long ago, an ACL rupture usually ended a player's career. It still does, sometimes. Anyway, we believed Paul's knee should heal with rest followed by rehab.

Although inconsistent, the team had some impressive results against the higher teams. The youngsters' team had won the FA Youth Cup in 1985 and Willie was fortunate to be able to call on some of those lads for the first team, such as Kevin Scott, Joe Allon and Ian Bogie. The precious gem among that gifted trophy-winning team had to be Gazza. He dazzled on the pitch, bewildering opponents with his movements, but then always knew when to deliver an inch-perfect pass, no matter how easy or difficult that was to do. Not only that, he was also extremely competitive and had a knack of winning most of his midfield tussles. Give him a chance on goal and the odds were he would score.

A good coach needs a good squad to be successful, and Willie was able to surround Gazza with a team to do the young star justice, from defensive stalwarts such as Glenn Roeder and John Anderson to ever-reliable David McCreery in midfield and, of course, the sublime star himself, Peter Beardsley. A special mention must go to Kenny Wharton, the utility player from Blakelaw, who always put in 100 per cent effort and added to the quality of the team. Although there was 'nowt' on Kenny, pound for pound he was one of the hardest players I worked with. With the steady captaincy of Glenn Roeder, the Toon finished in a respectable 11th place.

It was around this time that coach John Pickering heard the terrible news that his daughter was dying from leukaemia. As soon as the lads found out, they had a whip-round and got enough money together for John and his family to fly to Disney World in Florida.

Ferra had struggled with his fitness all season. Just when we thought he was ready to be injury-free, something broke down, either his knee or hamstring. I had my doubts about the stability of his knee. Willie packed him off on loan to Port Vale for the start of 1986/87, and I never saw him again … as a player.

Pre-season we went off to the Isle of Man tournament where, somehow, I manged to play up front with Peter Beardsley in a couple of the matches. We then went over to Northern Ireland for fixtures against Linfield and Coleraine to get ready for the new season. But 1986/87 didn't start well at all, and we were bottom after the turn of the year when we lost nine and drew one of ten matches. The signing of Paul Goddard proved to be crucial. His debut was in November, but he didn't start scoring regularly until February. Gazza returned from a groin strain and Paul Goddard went on a run of scoring in every match. We picked up valuable points in March and April, winning seven times. As the season approached its conclusion, we'd picked up enough points and finished in 17th place.

One match that stands out from this time was when we played West Ham away towards the end of April. They hammered us 8-1. We used three goalkeepers, and their centre-half Alvin Martin scored a hat-trick, netting against each of our three goalies. It has been called Newcastle's worst-ever goalkeeping display. To be fair, we started with Martin Thomas, who was already injured and had to come off at half-time. Centre-half Chris Hedworth started the second half in goal, then fractured his collarbone, so Peter Beardsley had to take over. The cherry on the cake must have been Glenn Roeder's comical backheel own goal.

Poor finances meant the board dictated the sale of Peter Beardsley to Liverpool before the start of the 1987/88 season. Although this was for a British record of £1.9m, surely he was worth more? Once again the team started the season poorly, losing two of the first three matches. The city was getting restless. The club signed Mirandinha as a replacement for Beardsley. This helped to temper the fans' frustration and the Brazilian's early performances established him as a favourite with the Toon army. Many of the fans, especially for the away matches, would proudly wear their sombreros in homage to Mira, their idol. They were particularly happy after he scored twice in the away draw with Man Utd in September. Things weren't looking so good a week later when Liverpool came to St James' and gave us a 4-1 hiding; Peter Beardsley was in their team and broke our hearts with his incredible skills.

A week later we had another home match, against Southampton. We won 2-1. By now Gazza was firmly established in the team, performing wonders, but still up to his antics. He loved nothing more than winding people up. At the beginning of October we went to London to play Chelsea and were staying at the Swallow International Hotel in Kensington before the match. The directors had met up with our London scout for some evening drinks. Gazza, being bored, was looking for something to do. First of all he had the girl on reception page 'Mike Hunt' for him. She paged Mike a couple of times, but there was no sign of him ... so Gazza was hanging about pestering her to page Mike Hunt again, and again. Then, somehow, he gained possession of our scout's wig. The hairpiece was a thing that we were all aware of, but were 'never to speak about', but somehow Gazza acquired it and attached a piece of fishing line to it. I have no idea how he had either the wig or the fishing line. So, this wig became an animated hairy entity on the polished floor in front of the hotel reception. Some unsuspecting guests would arrive to check in only to be scared witless by some 'thing' jerking its way across the floor towards them. Bless him, he never means any harm. The next day at Stamford Bridge we conceded two goals in the first half. In our recovery, Gazza was his wizardly best in the midfield, assisting in both of our goals in the 2-2 draw.

Willie signed Michael O'Neill in October. He combined well with Gazza. Teams were starting to fear the young lad from Dunston. Vinnie Jones's attempt to stop him was through intimidation. The famous photo of Vinnie grabbing Gascoigne's balls at Plough Lane was taken in February 1988. Straight after the match, when the teams were in the dressing rooms, Gazza sent Vinnie a rose and he returned the gesture, sending the teenager a bog brush. We thought nothing more of it until 'that' photo hit the front and back pages the following day.

Mira's input to the team had tailed off through the season, so we really benefitted from the way Gazza linked up with Michael O'Neill to supply him with scoring opportunities; the forward scored 12 goals in 19 matches in the run-in. As the season was nearing its end, we hammered Luton at home. They'd given our lads a hard time at Kenilworth Road, taking the piss, so Kenny Wharton decided to sit on the ball before Gazza did some showboating. The Hatters weren't happy, but revenge was sweet. We went on to finish a respectable eighth, winning our last three matches.

The final fixture was on Saturday, 7 May, then we had a friendly away at Whitley Bay on the Monday, for a testimonial.

John Anderson picked up a serious ankle injury, going over in a hole on the pitch. He'd ruptured his lateral ligament complex and the orthopaedic surgeon suspected that he had internal damage to the joint. As a result, Ando was put in a below-knee cast to enable the ligament to heal and minimise damage to the joint. This was particularly bad timing for him because he was hoping to play for Ireland in the Euro '88 championships in Germany. By this time, Jack Charlton had become established as the Ireland manager and his team had won through to the finals. So the injury meant no Euros for Ando. I was sitting at home one evening when he phoned me.

'Hello.'

'Hello, Derek. It's John.'

'Alright Ando. Everything okay?'

'I'm in Dublin, Derek.'

'Okay, you visitin' home?'

'No, I'm at the Ireland training camp.'

'What you there for?'

'I'm off to the Euros, Derek.'

'To watch?'

'No, to play.'

'What the …! You're in a plaster cast, man!'

'I took it off, so I did. Did the fitness test.'

'Did the *fitness* test? Don't tell me you passed it?'

'Aye, Jack just wanted to see me run in a straight line.'

So, that was that. Completely knackered ankle but off to the Euros. Whenever I see Ando now, hobbling about with his arthritic ankle, I remind him of that conversation!

* * *

Amid the open war between the rebel directors and the board, Willie was forced to sell Gazza to Spurs before the start of the new season; Paul Goddard and Neil McDonald were also sold. Paul Gascoigne, the lad from Dunston who three years earlier was carol singing for 20p bus fares was starting at Spurs on £2,500 a week. The new season started with a new chairman: Gordon McKeag; Willie was immediately under pressure. McKeag is infamous for referring to the club as 'the family silver', something some supporters wouldn't let him forget, complaining that the real family silver being sold was the promising group of star players, many of them Geordie lads who would give everything for the club and often went off to have stellar careers and achieve much greater financial value for other clubs. On a personal level, Mr McKeag was very kind to me; he always offering his support, as did the rest of the board.

Willie brought in useful players like John Hendrie and John Robertson, but we started the 1988/89 season poorly, losing 4-0 away to Everton. To make matters worse, Gazza was in the Spurs team for our first home match, which ended as a 2-2 draw. The crowd was merciless in its abuse of the lad. I think the message was, 'You are one of our own and you have betrayed us.' Losing great players like Waddle, Gascoigne and Beardsley in short order was bound to have a detrimental effect on the team's quality. One of Newcastle's tendencies over the years has been to sell off its best players too early.

When we lost 3-0 to Coventry at home on 8 October, Willie was sacked the following day. We'd played seven matches and had five points. I took it hard. It was my first experience of my manager being sacked, Malcolm and Jack having resigned. I felt bad for Willie and his family and confess that I shed tears. Having gone through that process once, I had to harden up to survive in the football world. Willie's assistant, Colin Suggett, took over from 9 October as caretaker while the board searched for a replacement.

Finally, Jim Smith started on 14 December 1988. By then we were bottom on 13 points and really missing Gazza in midfield.

My first son, Jonathan, was born in March, so I had my hands full for the rest of the season, watching my red-haired boy thriving, while helping Lisa and working. Having a family brings it home how difficult the world of professional football can be. I always ensured that I was at the training ground before the lads arrived, and I was usually the last to leave. I was responsible for all players, youth, reserve and first team. Most players who were in training left Benwell by early afternoon, but the injured players had to stay with me through the afternoon for their treatments or rehab training. All week I would be leaving the training ground at six o'clock or so, although I made sure I had every Sunday afternoon off.

Being the only physio, I covered all midweek and weekend fixtures. The reserves only played midweek. If there was an evening match I would be at Benwell through the day and went straight to St James' to prepare for the match. I would usually get home well after 11 o'clock, because, like the training ground, I was always the last to leave the players' changing room and coaches' room: one, to make sure everything was in order; and two, just in case a player returned with an issue, which they often did. Home matches at the weekend would mean arriving at the ground at least three hours before kick-off and leaving no sooner than two hours after the final whistle. Of course, away matches were another matter. A lot of preparation was necessary to ensure I had everything I needed. After that, timings were determined by travel arrangements. Sometimes for some of the closer fixtures, I would drive one of the players' cars back to the ground. Later on in my career, I travelled with Ray Thompson the kit man in the club van.

So, although I was home whenever I could be, my absences and being unable to help Lisa with Jonathan was a difficult juggling act. One way I had to deal with this was to make sure I was always around when my job permitted. It was only after I'd been at the club for five years that I persuaded General Manager Russell Cushing that I needed help covering reserve fixtures. I knew another physio who was working at the Queen Elizabeth Hospital in Gateshead, John Stevens. He was a very skilled sports physio and it was a great relief for me when he started to do the reserve matches.

* * *

The 1988/89 season continued to be a disaster; Jim tried some wheeling and dealing, bringing in keeper Tommy Wright and defender Kenny Sansom, but the team only picked up two points in the last nine matches. It was a slow exit from the top tier; we ended the campaign bottom and were relegated with 31 points. The attendance for the home defeat against West Ham was just under 14,500. The dark days had returned. No doubt about it, though, the darkest day for the whole country that season was the Hillsborough disaster on 15 April 1989. It certainly put our trials and tribulations into context.

In the close season, Jim took the team up to Peebles for some pre-season training. We were short of a left-back for one of the teams, so he asked me to fill in. He and his coach Bobby Saxton were talking to the lads while I was dealing with one of the players at the side of the pitch. *Here's my chance to impress*, I thought. The ball came out to me from Tommy Wright and we went to play it up the park. The ball went to the opposition, so I made a tackle, won the ball and played a one-two with Kenny Wharton. 'DEREK! DEREK! WHAT THE FUCK ARE YOU DOING? YOU STUPID TWAAAT!' I turned around to see, Jim Smith's face, puce with rage.

'Playing the ball up the wing,' I said.

'Playing t'fucking ball up t'fucking wing? Fucking listen to me! I said return the ball to Wrighty as soon as you lost the fucking thing.'

Half a dozen of the lads were standing behind him, sniggering. Well, that was the end of my potential Toon playing career. After the training he came up and put his arm around me, laughing: 'Fucking listen next time, son.'

Another memory of Jim I have was the late evenings sat up in hotels before away matches with him and his fellow-Yorkshireman Bobby Saxton. The night before a match I would be busy dealing with the lads, giving them massages, checking injuries and the like. Usually about 11 o'clock I would get a call to my room from Jim: 'Derek, get your arse down here, son. I'm talking to Bobby.' I would go down and join the two of them, downing two bottles of red wine and talking football. They really were very entertaining, regaling me with their colourful football stories. I could have done without the hangovers, though.

Before the start of 1989/90 in the Second Division, Smith brought in Micky Quinn and Mark McGhee, along with the experienced goalkeeper John Burridge. Mira was quietly sold by Jim back to his former club, Palmeiras. Micky scored four times in his home debut against Leeds, which we won 5-2. That developed into a good start for us, but the team wobbled in December. Off the pitch, the shares battle had built up again and there was some disquiet among the fans and in the press, although I always had the impression that Jim Smith was well liked. The fans' anger was always directed at the board while he was there. Amid the December defeats, Jim brought in Roy Aitken from Celtic. Roy was great in the centre of midfield and after a run of four 1-1 draws, we picked up a lot of wins from the end of February onwards.

My dad always came to the home matches. Mam would drop him off at the ground and afterwards I would take him home. I did it for decades. Afterwards, he would come down to the dressing room when most of the players had showered and gone to the players' lounge or headed home. I was usually tidying up or sorting a player in some way, so he would wait. Jim and Bobby always invited him into their coaches' room for a bit of crack and some wine. They never called him Derek, always 'Dad', because that's what I called him.

From the end of February we started winning regularly, but one of the rare defeats we had in that phase was away to Blackburn on 24 March 1990, but I remember it more for the 'fish and chips incident'. We did most of our away travelling by coach in those days. We had a tradition of buying fish and chips at the Wetherby Whaler on the way home. However, if we were playing at Blackburn, we used a local chippy. Another tradition in those days were doormen for the teams. These guys would stand outside the dressing rooms and anything the lads wanted, they would sort out, such as cups of tea or a snack. Anyway, we were at Ewood Park. My job was to give the order for the fish and chips to the doorman before the match so it would all be ready for the final whistle and the lads could eat them on the bus on the way home. I gave the order to the guy, something like ten fish and chips, half a dozen chicken and chips, pies, peas, etc. I gave the guy the order and I could tell from his glazed expression that he was struggling to understand. Eventually he went off with the money to get the order, hesitated, half turned but then left.

Not long after, Jim started the team talk, getting himself up into a tizzy as usual to get the lads going. Then came a knock on the door. Jim stopped and looked at me: 'Get the door, Derek.' I walked to the door. You could hear a pin drop. 'Please God, don't be the doorman with the chips order,' I said to myself. I opened the door. 'See the order, son; was it ten fish and chips or ten chicken and chips?'

'WHAT THE FUCKKK!!! Fish and fucking chips? Derek I'm trying to do t'fucking team talk here!' Jim shouted. I took doorman outside.

'Ten fish, six chicken, for fuck's sake.' I went back inside. Jim was still muttering 'fish and chips, chicken and chips' to himself. 'Anyway, Quinny, where was I?' Every fucker sniggering again. All good fun.

Micky Quinn *was* a scoring machine. He had that centre-forward's instinct for goal, being in the right place at the right time. Some fans argue that Quinny deserves to be in the Newcastle No. 9s' Hall of Fame. I certainly believe he's one of our great characters in that iconic shirt.

Things were looking very promising by mid-April, but the team slipped towards the end of the season. We finished third, just missing automatic promotion. Sunderland came sixth, taking the last play-off spot, meaning they would play us. The first play-off tie was away to the Mackems and we brought a 0-0 draw back to St James'. The expectation was that the home tie would be a formality, but Sunderland won 2-0. A pitch invasion by our supporters just added to the misery. That defeat was my worst experience in football up to that point. We thought we'd done the hard work by getting the away draw. Never assume anything in football.

I suppose that saying applies to life in general and not just football. About this time I was dealing with a young player with a serious neck fracture, Alan Thompson. Alan was just a 16-year-old schoolboy at the club when he could have died. He suffered a fracture dislocation of his cervical spine in a car accident on the way home from watching the reserves play at Leeds just as the new season was starting. When Doctor Beveridge and I heard of his injuries, our main concern was that he would never walk again, never mind become a professional footballer. He was extremely lucky not to be paralysed.

Alan needed a couple of operations and was required to wear a full plaster cast from his waist to his skull. Once we had to go-ahead from the surgeon, we had Alan on the static bike. His 17th birthday came and went but he just beavered away, always smiling and joking. Eventually the cast came off and we got into specific rehab for his neck while getting the rest of his physiology back to that of an athlete. To their credit, the club rewarded Alan with a pro contract, and he returned their faith in him by eventually achieving first-team status. Throughout his ordeal of about 14 or 15 months he never gave up and did not complain once.

We all had to put the disappointment of missing out on promotion behind us. The manager was very positive at the start of the 1990/91 season, but by March 1991 the team's performance was very inconsistent. We had a lot of injuries to deal with. Jim Smith had been trying to bring in one or two expensive signings, but the board was having nothing to do with that, and he resigned in frustration. This was amid the power struggle and shares battle that by this point had reached board level. Newcastle United FC was still controlled by the original directors at this point, in particular the McKeag and Seymour families. The chairman, Gordon McKeag, was a Newcastle solicitor who inherited a boardroom seat at the club when his father died in 1972. He became chairman in 1988. The Magpie Group, in trying to take control away from them, had managed to get John Hall a seat on the board. He'd made his money in property development and his current project was the Metro Centre. In the eyes of the supporters he was what they wanted: originally from Ashington mining stock, but with the financial clout to change the club's fortune.

Clandestine meetings had been taking place with some board members to see if any were prepared to help. Shares were purchased whenever possible from anyone willing to sell. Those of the Geordie diaspora who owned shares were visited in various parts of the country by representatives of the rebels and offered good money for their shares. Once the Magpie Group had 40 per cent of the shares, the club had to allow John on the board. As shares changed hands, he brought his son, Douglas, and Freddy Shepherd and Freddie Fletcher alongside him under the Cameron Hall Developments banner. Meanwhile, McKeag was doing everything he could to maintain control, short of putting funds into the squad. As part of the struggle, John Hall forced a public share issue, but that flopped. The supporters had no trust in the board while the original directors were still in charge; they'd been given enough time to achieve success but had failed. Nevertheless, John Hall had become the figurehead for the rebels, supported by many determined individuals, not least Malcolm Dix and some of the original Magpie Group.

It was amid this rancour that Jim Smith went. The power struggle was unprecedented and continued after he left. Fans expressed their displeasure with the way the club was being run, while journalists including Bob Cass and John Gibson made it clear that newspapers such as the *Evening Chronicle* were in favour of change. It was actual potential bankruptcy that forced the change; the bank had withdrawn overdraft support and called in a loan when it was used inappropriately, no doubt because the incumbents were desperate to buy players and effect change on the pitch. There was only one man in the city at that time who was able to bail out the club, and that was John Hall. It was only a matter of time until his group had sufficient shares for him to gain ownership.

Jim Smith was replaced by Ossie Ardiles. Ossie was appointed in March 1991. I found him to be a very warm and approachable man. His coach was Tony Galvin, who was academically bright. I believe he had a degree in Russian, which isn't something you see in football every day. My impression was that between them they were astute tacticians. We finished the season in 11th place. Not bad for the first tier but we were second tier. Ossie had the ability to turn it around, but he needed the support of the new board.

I turned out for a Newcastle XI at a testimonial at Whitley Bay during the close season. That was a good laugh, but it marked the last time I ever pulled on the shirt for any representative match. Oh, well. It didn't stop me having vivid dreams that I was needed in the team and of running out at St James'… I wonder how many other supporters have had similar ones. It was around this time that I developed the habit of racing the opposition's physio on to the pitch. It's surprising how often we both need to come on at the same time. I would sometimes notice the other physio trying a bit too hard, so I thought, *Bugger that, there's no way they're beating me.* From then on it was a race. It was one of the home matches against Charlton that I noticed the crowd cheering, so it became a regular thing. Once Darren Peacock even blocked the opponents' physio's path to make sure he didn't beat me. I broke my foot (again) some years later, and that put paid to those antics.

The club celebrated its change in name to Newcastle United in the centenary season of 1991/92. We started the campaign with a lot of hope, but our start was patchy and before long we were struggling. We drew too many matches, and the victories were infrequent. It was a difficult time. There was no money available for new players and we relied heavily on youngsters. Several of these lads went on to have great careers, but with such a young team it was a struggle competing at this level. We did have some very good senior players at that time, though: Quinny, Roy Aitken and Mark McGee as examples. Ossie gave Alan Thompson his debut in November after he finally recovered from his horror crash, but we were still losing or drawing too many times.

Although I knew nothing of the club's politics other than newspaper articles, at board level the battles continued. McKeag had handed over the chairmanship to Borders farmer George Forbes. Before Christmas, Sir John Hall (he was knighted in the 1991 Birthday Honours) had acquired sufficient shares to become the largest individual shareholder. McKeag and Russell Cushing lost their seats on the board. The Cameron Hall enterprise was taking control and it was only a matter of time until Sir John replaced George as chairman.

Sir John was supportive of Ossie initially, but he wasn't as popular with some of the new board members, and they made the decision to sack Ossie. Although Sir John had a good personal relationship with the Argentine, he sensed that the club was going nowhere. He might have kept going with him, but the other Cameron Hall directors were pushing for change. Ossie was sacked on 5 February 1992. It was a sad moment for me, as Ossie was a considerate manager with a jocular personality away from the cameras, and he had the respect of the players. In many ways, the period leading up to Ossie's departure was pivotal in the club's history. The two-year boardroom struggle was over and a new owner was in control, an owner with passion but also big pockets. But weren't we happy when we heard of Ossie's replacement: none other than local hero, Kevin Keegan!

Chapter 4

Keegan Returns

ALMOST EIGHT years after King Kev flew out of St James'
in the helicopter to the waves of an eternally grateful Geordie
crowd, including an inconspicuous 13-year-old ball boy called
Alan Shearer, he returned as manager. He was my sixth manager
in under eight years. The club ascended to a new level the day
he returned. Kevin had been out of professional football since
that emotional day on 17 May 1984. He'd spent most of that
time in Spain but had recently returned to live in Hampshire.
A couple of charity events had brought him back to Tyneside.
While in the region, he'd been sounded out for paid engagements
related to the club's centenary by chairman George Forbes and
vice-chairman Peter Mallinger. That role fell through, allegedly
on Ossie's insistence.

Next, he was approached by the 'rebels' on the board and
asked to take over as manager. He met with Freddie Fletcher,
Freddy Shepherd, Sir John Hall and Douglas Hall in London on
Monday, 3 February 1992. Once Kevin had assurances about funds
for players, he agreed to take the job. He knew that Sir John was
less enthusiastic about the appointment than his Cameron Hall
colleagues. As he put it in his autobiography, it must have been the
first time in football history that a manager had been appointed

without the knowledge of the chairman or vice-chairman, and the future chairman didn't want him!

Of course, we knew nothing about this until the press announcement. In general, players and staff alike hear very little about what goes on at boardroom level. The two parts of the club are quite distinct, and that separation has increased over the years; I only know Newcastle United, but I suspect that's the case in most clubs. Still, it was a shock to hear that Ossie was on his way out the door, but with the news that King Kev was returning, the city was buzzing. Every time a new manager is appointed a little voice suggests you might be walking out through the revolving door that the manager's entering with his own staff. Fortunately, back in the early 90s this was unusual, and I knew Kevin had been out of the game for eight years so it would be unlikely that he had another physio in mind.

In my opinion, the decision he made to bring Terry McDermott in with him was genius. Terry had been training with the team after his contract expired but, when Arthur Cox resigned, Big Jack kicked him out. To be more specific, the club had retained Terry's registration and Jack expected him to sign on the same contract he had while playing alongside Kevin in the promotion team. Terry believed he should have an improved contract and Jack told him to come back when he was ready to sign his old contract. He never went back, as a player. He was selling burgers at Liverpool racetracks to make a living when Kev called him. He valued Terry Mac's presence so much that he paid his salary from his own pocket. Another very important appointment was Derek Fazackerley as first-team coach. Faz was a *great* coach. He was the organiser, tactician and planner for Kevin. With the framework provided by Faz, Kevin and Terry were able to construct the attacking team they required. Their skill was to identify subtle areas in the team that needed work, either through one-on-one coaching or drills. There was no better man-manager than Kevin.

To Kevin's credit, one of the first things he ordered was a repair and paint job at the training ground. It had become increasingly neglected since I arrived, despite my frequent requests to the Russell Cushing to have it cleaned and repaired. I'm sure Russell's requests to the directors fell on deaf ears. When Kevin insisted, it was a done deal.

The first time I had a meeting with Kevin, he came across as very approachable, but he said he was minded to send any players who had ongoing problems down to Fred Street, who could see them in the Park Street private clinic in London. I was taken aback by this. I explained that I had a lot of respect for Fred, knowing him personally, but suggested that using him would not be necessary. I asked Kevin to wait and see how we got on with the injuries. After that we never needed to send anyone down to see Fred.

Kevin Keegan was an inspirational manager, never coming across as authoritarian at all, and Terry's bubbly personality was a great foil to Kevin's leadership. For me, the theme for the whole time Kevin was manager was one of unstoppable invincibility. There was always the winning expectation. I never had that feeling for such a long period of time with any other manager. He always got 100 per cent out of his staff and players anyway, but between manager and assistant they never missed a trick and there was no corner-cutting with them. Nothing got past Terry, and if Terry knew it, Kevin knew it. Terry became known as Kevin's 'buffer'. Everything had to go through Terry first. Having said that, they both gave their full commitment as well. They're the only bosses who would come to the ground for every away match with Ray Thompson and me and help us unload the skips containing the kit and equipment. They would then take a wander out to the pitch and take in the surroundings. If there were any pre-match fitness tests I needed to do, Kevin would watch the proceedings. He always listened to my suggestions and never went against any absolutes, but if there was any room for coaxing players into playing, he would be there with his arm around them, letting them know how vital they were.

* * *

Kevin Keegan has very strong links to the North East, and Stanley itself. His dad was born in Hetton-le-Hole and grew up there, moving to Donny like many miners did, to find work in the Doncaster coalfield. Kevin's grandfather, Frank, was a pit inspector in the West Stanley Colliery on the afternoon of 16 February 1909 when one of the worst pit disasters in UK history occurred. Frank was below ground when there was an issue with two fuses blowing in the generator house on the surface. Five minutes later there was a small explosion below ground, followed some seconds later by a massive explosion that caused flames to burst out of one of the shafts, followed by plumes of black smoke. Only moments later the asphyxiating cloud was sucked back down the shaft, leaving fresh air at the surface. Both shafts were damaged, and it took some time for rescuers to get down 'inbye'. Tragically, 186 men and boys died, some as young as 13. That's the same as the number of dots on a set of dominoes.

The two shafts went through eight seams. The explosion occurred in the second-deepest level, the busty seam. The pit was known to have problems with excessive coal dust. Once coal dust is ignited, it will explode because of the very large surface area relative to the size of the particles. None other than Michael Faraday himself, the inventor of the electric motor, had worked that out after visiting the scene of another explosion in a County Durham pit about 50 years earlier.

An electrical spark is likely to have ignited a pocket of firedamp (methane gas), which then exploded the coal dust. The shock wave precedes the flame; this lifts coal dust off everything, suspending it in air, waiting to be ignited by the flame. The miners would have died as a direct result of the explosion, or asphyxia because all the oxygen is consumed by the fire. If a lot of methane is present, afterdamp is also formed (carbon monoxide). What an insidious gas carbon monoxide is: it grabs on to the blood cells like a clamp, displacing oxygen, and won't let go. Frank Keegan was one of the lucky survivors, but he was trapped below ground and immediately helped with the rescue effort. He continued even after *his* rescuers arrived several hours later. He and Joseph Snaith were awarded a gold medal for bravery. I know that Kevin is proud of his grandfather's actions that day.

* * *

On the football pitch, Kevin's first match as manager was the 3-0 victory over Bristol City. He said in his book that he'd been out of the game so long that all he knew about their opponents was that they played in red. Of course, Kevin's presence changed the atmosphere in the city completely: it went from despair to hope and excitement. What's more, this gave the board the breathing space required to complete their restructure, with Sir John formally taking over as chairman. There was a slight hiccup early on when Kevin almost left the club because of a dispute with Sir John over funding for players, but once that was sorted Kevin steadied the ship. He brought in 6ft 4in Brian Kilcline to join another couple of older pros, Liam O'Brien and Franz Carr, that he and Terry Mac could rely on. Meanwhile, yet another batch of young talent from the North East was beginning to impress on the training field. Steve Watson and Lee Clark would run all day, and showed immense promise, while big Steve Howey was about to discover that he would make a much better centre-half than centre-forward. And then we had the likes of Alan Thompson and Robbie Elliott. It's unlikely that we'll ever see as many Geordies in the team as back then.

We won a few matches and moved up the league. Terry started talking about a play-off place, but we then immediately lost 6-2 away to Wolves and lost the next four in a row! The club was staring at the Third Division for the first time in its history. It came down to the last two matches and a breathless end to the season befitting of Kevin's tenure. We won the first of those at home against Portsmouth with a David ('Ned') Kelly goal five minutes from time. In the final match away to Leicester City, a last-minute own goal by Steve Walsh just after he'd equalised confirmed our place in the Second Division for next season. I witnessed my third major pitch invasion as a physio. This time the Leicester fans went on, first when they thought they'd secured a draw, and then in despair when Walsh passed the ball past his own keeper into the empty net. They tried to antagonise the Newcastle supporters, separated by a line of police. Both sets of fans squared up, sandwiching the police, so the referee made the decision that the match had ended. That was that, unlike the Fulham match at Derby, the decision by the referee at the time meant it was all over, and the Toon were safe.

Towards the end of the season, Kevin brought in a part-time fitness coach, Steve Black. I would describe Blackie as a working-class polymath. He grew up on a council estate in Benton, left school at the earliest opportunity and started working as a trainee accountant. In his spare time he combined a passion for sport and coaching, which resulted in him running all sorts of teams and fitness classes from elite amateurs to over 65s. He also loved a fight and I'm told he was very good at it, so he was invited to be a nightclub doorman and had become a very well-known bouncer and employer of bouncers. That was his evening job. Prior to being recommended to Kevin, Steve had undertaken a degree in sports studies at Newcastle Polytechnic (later renamed as Northumbria University).

Although Blackie had great knowledge and ability as a fitness coach, it was his sports psychology that was valued in Kevin's set-up. He'd realised very early on that psychology was massively important in achieving the best results in sport. He was able to work very well with Faz to produce impressive results. To start with, on the physical side at training, Blackie would help Faz by taking the lads for warm-up, getting them into the right frame of mind for the session, then take them for the warm-down. As time passed, he would also do one-on-one chats with players who needed it. He also introduced a weight-training programme. Not all players needed the additional strength training, but Blackie was years before his time in being able to look at players as individuals and work out what they needed to supplement their training, be that additional strength, flexibility or cardiovascular fitness.

Over the summer we all expected Kevin and Terry to stay on and ride the crest of the wave; however, there were nagging rumours that Kevin had resigned. As it turned out, he hadn't signed a contract to resign *from*, and when he met with the directors it was apparent that money would not be forthcoming. He went off to Spain. Behind the scenes, the power struggle finally tipped with the share balance when director Bob Young sold his shares. This forced other directors to sell theirs, giving Sir John the share majority as an individual. This was another of those moments that changed Newcastle United that most of us had no idea about. So, with renewed promises from Sir John, Kevin finally signed a manager's contract and Terry got his assistant manager's contract too.

Chapter 5

1992–1994

WHEN THE new season started, the boardroom was completely controlled by the Cameron Hall empire, led by the owner Sir John and supported by his son, Douglas, and Freddy Shepherd. The Toon were now in the First Division, but only because the new Premier League had been created and the second tier had been renamed. A massive bonus for all the staff was our move to the Maiden Castle training ground in Durham. We had to share the facilities with the university students, but that wasn't a problem and, besides, the playing surfaces were immaculate.

We won the first 11 matches, starting with an away win at Southend. The team showed the flare that was to become a hallmark of the Keegan period. Lee Clark (Nash) was ever-present and captain Brian Kilcline (Killer) marshalled the team brilliantly. It helped that Killer was a very likeable guy and he certainly helped to brighten up every day at the training ground. Steve Howey was also proving to be a superb centre-half under Killer's tutelage. In goal, Pavel Srníček, who had been a Jim Smith signing, established himself as first-choice keeper. Kevin brought in top-drawer pros in Barry Venison, John Beresford and Paul Bracewell.

Paul Bracewell's appointment was interesting. Both of his ankles were significantly 'shot', for want of a better word.

He'd suffered repeated injuries and was showing signs of early osteoarthritis. He'd just turned 30, and with those ankles I knew it was a significant risk to sign him. I told Kevin that should I do a formal medical on him, I would have to fail him on the condition of his ankles. Kevin came straight back to me: 'Don't do a medical on him then. He played over forty games for Sunderland last season.' So that was that, he would have had a medical of sorts but we accepted that he had old man's ankles. Paul turned out to be a trooper. He was one of more important players that season and we managed his ankles carefully before and after every match with strapping and ice packs, and he got through it. I respected Kevin for his decision; he knew Paul's ankles were a mess but he also knew he was somehow able to put in top-class performances despite that.

Barry (Venna) had gone to my old school in Stanley (as did Brian Tinnion and then the Miley brothers many years later) and I'd played a few times with his dad, Davey, for East Stanley Working Men's Club, so that was a nice connection. Like father, like son: Davey and Barry, both 'radgie as'. Rob Lee arrived in September. He turned out to be one of Kevin's most important signings. Famously, Kevin persuaded him to choose the Toon over Boro because Newcastle 'was closer', according to Kev. Early in his time with us, Rob Lee was recovering from an ankle sprain. I did his 20-minute fitness test, which he managed fine other than struggling a bit to cross a ball in from the right side. I told Kevin this. 'That's great, Derek,' he said. 'I'll play him on the left. Rob, you okay starting on the left?' 'Yes, boss. No problem,' Rob replied. So that was that! Rob played on the left and did fine.

Not long after Rob Lee arrived, Kevin sold Micky Quinn to Coventry. Micky tells a story that he would play, score a goal or two and Kevin would drop him. He would pick him again, Micky would score, only to be dropped for the next match. He'd finally had enough and went to see Kevin, telling him that he wanted to know his future because he didn't know if he was 'coming or going'. Kevin replied, 'Well, I can answer that for you, Quinny: you're going. I've just accepted an offer for you from Bobby Gould at Coventry so get yer bags packed!'

In February 1993 Kevin broke the club's transfer record to bring in Andy Cole. At the time he was unknown to most people. He was a quiet lad, always polite and considerate. He told me early on that he preferred to be called Andrew, so I tried to remember to call him that as I have from here on. Nash raved about him because of his experience of training and playing with him for England Schoolboys.

The supporters were allowed to attend the training sessions at Maiden Castle, which was fantastic for them. It allowed the diehards the opportunity to get closer to their idols. Sometimes over 5,000 attended a training session. It was a real party atmosphere. What was slightly bizarre was most of the changing facilities were shared with the students. Not that it was ever a problem. I think *they* had the greater problem because their lovely training facilities had been invaded by hordes of Geordie football supporters! Some of my fondest memories working for the club were from the time we were in Durham. It was one of the golden periods. You must remember this was before mobile phones. The players could get away with saying things and larking about that would today inevitably be videoed and immediately put on YouTube or TikTok.

It was during one of those early summer training sessions when we were heading for promotion that Arthur had one of his 'wise old owl' moments. The lads were wrapping up training, Kevin and Terry were in one of their famous head tennis games, arguing melodramatically about a point. 'Savour this son,' Arthur said. 'These are special times, they might never come again.' He was right, they were special times that none involved would ever forget. Things just got better, and we came from 1-0 down away to Millwall to win 2-1, then beat the Mackems 1-0 at St James' when Scott Sellars scored with a well-worked free kick early on. But, wow! The Millwall supporters are brutal. For the away fixture, I had to attend to one of our players near the far corner so had to walk back around the goal to the dugout. It was the Old Den, about three weeks before their last match there. The fans were caged in but very close to the track. They all had a go as I walked back: 'Facking Geordie Caann' ... Look at you, you facking fat bastard! Geordie CAANN'!' All the way back to the dugout. Ray Thompson was killing himself. 'Fuck's sake, Tommo, I hope I don't have to do that again.'

One of the high points of my career was just over two weeks after the Sunderland win. The season was nearly over, and it was a Tuesday evening, 4 May 1993. We were playing Grimsby down at Cleethorpes. About a third of the ground had Newcastle supporters packed inside. There were still two matches left after this one, but if we won here we knew we were promoted. Just after the start of the second half, Andrew scored a classic 'Andy Cole' goal, put through by Rob Lee and calmly passing past the advancing keeper. Ned Kelly then finished them off in the 90th minute when he took it round the keeper, stumbled but regained his balance and slotted it neatly inside the post. When the ref blew the final whistle, a lot of pent-up emotion was released, and the Toon fans invaded the pitch. This was the fourth major pitch invasion of my career, but by far the happiest.

The lads ran into the dressing room as the Grimsby supporters streamed out of the ground, but the Newcastle supporters wouldn't leave so we went out and did a lap of honour, which was just a big party down in the goalmouth with our supporters. Mickey Holland, who was later to become our masseur, was there as a fan wearing a Batman outfit. He placed a plastic crown on Kevin's head: 'King' Kevin. That became an iconic image. I remember a fan rushed up to me: 'How, Wrighty. I went to school with yous! Year below.' Before I could say anything, he was gone in the melee and the rumpus, in the confusion that continued for another ten minutes or so until the security and police politely suggested it was time for everyone to go home. What a night!

We played Oxford at home on the Thursday evening just two days after the Grimsby match. It was 0-0 at half-time. Kevin was pissed off, saying there had been too much partying. He threatened to go home if the performance didn't improve. We eventually won 2-1, but when the lads came in, Kev had gone! He was at St James' three days later for the last match, which finished our fourth consecutive season in the lower tier. It was against Leicester. The match was very different to the equivalent one against the same opposition the preceding year. This time we were already champions, and we hammered our opponents 7-1 in front of our home crowd. We finished eight points clear. That was the game Pav showed off his 'Pavel is a Geordie' T-shirt while doing the lap of honour. The people of Newcastle always afforded him that accolade from that day onwards. Andrew Cole and David Kelly both scored hat-tricks. For Andrew that was 12 goals in 12 matches. David did extremely well for the Toon, and people sometimes forget how important he was. He scored 39 goals in 83 appearances, but the Leicester match was the last he played for us. Kevin sold him to Wolves; he was always looking to upgrade the team.

There was a big party in Newcastle the night we were promoted. I ended up dancing in a skip with Ray Thompson in China Town in the early hours. There were similar scenes all over the city. This was a period of intense 'Geordie pride' (isn't it always?). Sir John Hall had expressed a desire to have as many Geordies as possible playing in the team. This begs the questions: what is a Geordie, and where can a Geordie come from? Tony Toward, the team operations manager, would often tell me that he was a Geordie because he was born in Newcastle, but I wasn't because I was born in Stanley. He was always very specific: 'Born in Hopedean Maternity Hospital on Elswick Road, Derek. Within a mile of the Tyne!' Much has been written about what qualifies a person as a Geordie, but it really has to do with who used the Stephenson ('Geordie') lamp down the pit. So, basically most places in the region that had mines and miners were likely to use the local lamp, called the Geordie lamp, and these lads spoke pitmatic, which is a version of the North East accent strongly associated with the Geordie identity. However, no one should feel excluded; being a Geordie today is to do with social class, accent and feeling part of the region. It's also a very inclusive club: anyone can join!

* * *

With promotion under Kev, the clamour for season tickets locally as well as rising attention nationally meant they had to modernise everything, and fast. This meant improving a range of things, from increasing the number of admin staff to deal with ticketing issues to sorting out the training facilities and developing the dilapidated stadium. The Sir John Hall Stand went up over the summer. Our medical department needed to modernise as well. I had no first-team physiotherapy assistant, and I was still doing the daily work and covering the first-team matches at weekends and evenings.

I had Dr Keith Beveridge to call on as my medical support, but he was still a full-time GP working in Sedgefield and

Fishburn. He was such a great person and a well-respected doctor. His support in the early days had been invaluable and he'd welcomed me into his home and family with his wife June and his two boys Neil and Mark. The doc did his best to persuade the club to bring in colleagues, but his requests had been fruitless. I told Kevin and Terry Mac that we really needed another physio, and when Keith backed me up they didn't need any more persuasion, so Russell Cushing had to agree to the club finding the additional salary.

I'd bumped into Paul Ferris, Ferra, a couple of times when I was covering reserve fixtures. He told me he was now a student physio at the uni in Newcastle. Out of the blue he sent me his final year thesis: 'The Role of the Physiotherapist in Professional Football.' I was really impressed by his wordsmanship and as he was from a football pedigree, having progressed much further in the game as a player than I had, I took notice. Ferra used to hold the record of being the youngest debutant for the club, but Steve Watson had just broken it. One statistic that jumped out at me from his thesis was that 80 per cent of physios in professional football at that time were unqualified. I knew that Paul was the physio I wanted, but I had to wait.

* * *

I must mention the 'Ayia Napa incident', which happened over the summer after the 1992/93 season. As a bit of a celebration, some of the lads went off to Nissi beach, Cyprus, for a long weekend, being 'looked after' by Derek Fazackerley, the coach. They all got smashed, of course. The incident then happened: Brian Kilcline, while fast asleep, had his ponytail cut off and half his tash shaved. Killer's lion's mane and facial hair were his pride and joy. I think it's fair to say after all these years that the consensus is Barry Venison was the culprit ... but was it also Faz? It's still openly debated whether Faz had more than a passive role in the incident. Killer was unconscious with the drink when the deed was done. Some hours later, when he discovered what happened, he went crazy. He thought it was one of the young lads, Alan Thompson, Steve Watson, Lee Clark or Robbie Elliot. When he was hunting them down, Faz tried to calm him and took a punch for his troubles. Amid the melee, lads were bouncing off him like bowling pins, but he eventually calmed down.

The supposed culprit didn't own up at the time, I think for good reason. Venna could be a bit of a wild lad when he had a few drinks in him. As I said, I knew his dad, Davey. He was a Stanley miner and, although well into his 40s, was still playing football himself at the time. Venna could get quite argumentative when the mood took him. I'm not sure how good he was at taking it though ... He loved his hair, did Venna. We were going on a night out not long after that and he got into the back of the taxi beside me. His hair looked so good, I put him in a headlock and gave his coiffure a proper scraggin'. He was so upset with me that he got out the taxi and went home! He didn't speak to me until I apologised.

We started 1993/94 with eager anticipation. Kevin brought Peter Beardsley back from Liverpool, for £1.35m at the age of 31. Peter was looking at a move to Derby, but Kevin convinced Sir John that his target was going to sign for the Mackems, so the chairman hurriedly found the money to bring the local hero back to Tyneside. We started with two defeats, the first at home to Spurs in front of the new Leazes End stand, which had been an uncovered terrace since the old stand was demolished in 1978. The third match was away to Man Utd. Kevin had already warned Sir Alex that the Toon were after their title; the Glaswegian would have responded gleefully to that threat through the media if we'd lost. We managed to get a draw thanks to an Andrew Cole goal, and we were up and running.

It might have been when we were away for this match that Terry Mac said something he wished he hadn't. Before I say it, I must say that footballers in the 1990s were not 'PC'. Are they now? Also, Terry always gave as good as he got, but on the night before the match he came into the hotel lounge to announce to a group of players and staff: 'Soup and sandwiches at six o'clock.' Terry has a bit of a lisp, so it came out as, 'Shoup and shandwiches at shix.' To this day, he's still reminded of that.

Shortly after the trip to Manchester, I contacted Paul Ferris; the doc and I had an informal interview with him. Once again, he impressed, so we offered him the job as assistant physio. He handed in his notice at the Freeman Hospital the next day. He couldn't have wished to start in this role at a better time. It must have been an omen, because we went on to win the next four matches, including a breathless 3-0 defeat of Liverpool at St James'. As the season progressed, Cole was on fire, seemingly scoring at will.

We were then witnesses to a brilliant virtuoso performance when we came up against Southampton at The Dell in October. Matt Le Tissier had been dropped for five matches before being recalled against us. Based on our performance, we should have won that day, but Le Tissier scored two wonder goals. First, he received a pass by flicking a backheel, then lobbed the ball over Venna, followed by another lob over Scott Sellars before side-footing it past Mike Hooper. For the second he teed up another pass with his thigh outside the box and volleyed the ball into the top right corner. We lost 2-1. That was the day Nash reacted when Kevin brought him off. Pissed off, he took it out on my kit bag by hoofing it when the manager chased after him down the tunnel and told him to sit on the bench. It didn't bother me, but Kevin wasn't impressed. After the match, Kevin gave the lads a right bollocking.

Andrew and Nash were good mates from way back in the England Schoolboy days. Andrew has gone on record to say that he didn't like the way Kevin treated his mate that time. We had a League Cup tie away at Wimbledon three days later. Kevin felt Andrew was putting in less effort during training down in London, which culminated in an exchange on the training pitch. I'm not sure whether Andrew was trying to make a point on behalf of his team-mate, but the boss wasn't the sort of bloke to mess with. Kevin invited him to 'fuck off' if he wasn't interested, and that's what he did … for three days! He missed the Wimbledon match, which we lost 2-1. Nash was dropped but Andrew was AWOL. He eventually came back and apologised. To his credit, he ended the season with impressive statistics, but I suspect Kevin never forgot that episode.

There was another unusual combination of events that involved Wimbledon again, not long after Andrew's disappearance. This time it started away to Luton in an FA Cup replay on Wednesday, 9 February 1994, which we lost 2-0. We had a league match against Wimbledon on the Saturday, so Kevin decided to keep the lads down south. We were in a hotel in Bournemouth, the Royal Bath Hotel. Andrew hurt his shoulder in the match at Kenilworth Road, so I had to spend some time in London with him getting X-rays and seeing a specialist. When we got down to Bournemouth the next day, I met Ray Thompson in the foyer of the hotel. Tommo looked shaken. Arthur Cox had already quizzed him about a suspicious empty bottle of champagne he saw on the Thursday morning. 'Raymond, who is in room 125?' he asked. Tommo checked the manifest.

'Steve Howey. Why?'

'There's an empty bottle of champagne outside it.'

Quick as lightening, Tommo replied, 'Yes, but anyone could have left that there.'

'Agreed,' Arthur said. 'Interesting though.'

There was a match coming up, so the lads had been forbidden any drinking sessions, but Venna, Steve Howey and Alex Mathie had decided to sneak out to one of the local bars. They might have gotten away with it, but Kevin and Terry had booked a laser-shooting outing in the afternoon for the lads, starting at 2pm. When those three went missing, Kevin went down to the taxi rank outside, asked if any of them had taken any players anywhere, and he and Terry were immediately taken to the wine bar they were drinking in. The three of them were despatched back to the hotel and were disciplined, but it didn't end there. After the laser afternoon, some more of the lads had beers in the hotel. Nash had a reputation for wearing his heart on his sleeve. In particular, he hated with a passion being dropped. As the drink flowed, he'd been bouncing around the lounge bar with Watto, enjoying himself, but something triggered Nash, and when Kevin arrived he let him have it with both barrels. This was one of those events that Kevin let go like water off a duck's back. Sometimes it's not worth the hassle. Nash was taken to his room. We then went up to Wimbledon for the match on Saturday and lost that 4-2. This was the John Fashanu and Vinnie Jones era. They battered and bullied the lads that day. Most of those involved in the Bournemouth shenanigans played. Kevin didn't say anything after the match; he didn't need to!

Nevertheless, Andrew became one of Newcastle's legendary No. 9s that season. He scored a hat-trick in our 4-0 defeat of Coventry at St James' in February; that got us started on a tremendous run and we ended up finishing in third place, qualifying for Europe.

The fans started to come to matches expecting a win as well as exciting football. It was the time the team were referred to as 'The Entertainers' by one or two journalists. Then Sky referred to them as that too. Andrew broke the club record for the number of goals scored in a season (all competitions), when he reached 41 in 45 matches. Prior to that, Hughie Gallacher and George Robledo shared that honour (Hughie scored 39 in 41 league and cup appearances in 1926/27 and George scored 39 in 47 league and cup appearances in 1951/52, although Hughie still holds the record for *league* goals: 36 in 38 matches in the same 1926/27 season). But it wasn't just about Andrew Cole. Peter Beardsley scored 24 times as well, and the pair of them playing together were brilliant to watch. Rob Lee was showing his class, too. We weren't conceding many either, and the fans had taken Pavel Srníček to their hearts.

Arthur was a great addition to the coaching staff. I can understand why Kevin decided to bring him back into the set-up after he'd worked under him as a player. Faz was a brilliant coach in all respects, but it was becoming a bit of a handful down at Maiden Castle with the public access and demands placed of the staff and players for the team to reach peak playing performance, so having Arthur there was a big help to Faz. Both men are still close friends of mine and I keep in regular contact with them. Arthur has been described as a 'sergeant major' type. I don't see him like that, but the very first away match I did with him, he asked me what time we were meeting for the pre-match meal. 'Eleven forty-five, I presume,' I said. He looked at me, shocked.

'Presume ...? *Presume? Never* presume, son.' So, that was me told, I made sure I never presumed anything with Arthur after that. He must have thought I was okay because we became good friends and reliable work colleagues. I helped him rehab after a meniscectomy (knee cartilage operation) and he was always grateful for that. Early on in his spell working under Kevin, before a match he put two tots of brandy into my and Tommo's coffees to go with his. 'Get that inside yous, boys,' he said. We went on to win, so after that it became a bit of a superstition/tradition that he had to put brandy tots in our coffees before each match.

If there was ever anything that escaped Terry, Arthur would notice it. One day we were about to start the team talk for a Sunday afternoon home match. Ray Thomson, Tommo, was sorting out the players' kits, but was struggling; he'd badly sprained his ankle playing football for a pub team, Scotswood Social, in the morning and was hobbling about trying not to be noticed. Earlier, Arthur had asked me what was up with 'Raymond', so I told him. Tommo was standing in the treatment room, hiding behind me and Ferra when Kevin started his team talk. All the players were seated around the benches beside the walls. 'Just before we start, lads ... Ray! Come here, will you pal?' Tommo scurried forwards, limping heavily. He then had to hop into the middle of the room. 'Got a problem with your ankle?'

'Aye, sprained it.'

'How'd ye do that?'

'Playin' football.'

'When?'

'This mornin'.'

Kevin then proceeded to rip into Tommo, telling him that he always needed 100 per cent commitment from *all* staff. He absolutely battered the poor lad. Tommo packed in his Sunday morning football after that! First thing the next day, Kevin organised for him to have his ankle X-rayed at the Nuffield private hospital.

Before the start of the 1994/95 season we had another trip to Ayia Napa, a reward for finishing third. This was for five days. In hindsight, perhaps a party central resort in the middle of summer for young British footballers in the 90s wasn't a great idea. The lads had drunk the plane dry by the time it arrived in Cyprus. Alex Mathie fell down the stairs getting off the plane. Robbie Elliot had had surgery on his knee and had his leg in a cast. The lads went straight from the hotel to the nearest bar. Meanwhile, Steve Watson, who wasn't drinking, had taken himself off somewhere. I thought he was being sensible and had gone for a walk. Robbie managed to fall off his bar stool and cut his leg on broken glass. I helped him back up and tried to lecture him about looking after his knee. I went up to the bar to get the round in. When I returned, I noticed Robbie had disappeared. I walked out on the terrace to see if he was out there. Some idiot was racing up and down the street on one of those mopeds. I was just about to go back inside when the bike came by again. 'DEERREEKK!' someone shouted. It sounded like Robbie. The rider of the moped started beeping its tinny horn. *WTF*, I thought. Then I saw them, Watto shirtless and helmetless driving, Robbie pillion with his knackered leg sticking out at 45 degrees from the bike. It took me two weeks to recover from that trip.

Chapter 6

1994–1995

THE 1994/95 season started brilliantly. We won our first six matches and went top. It was about this time we noticed that Newcastle were becoming people's second club because of the style of play. We didn't lose until the end of October. That was away to Man Utd. In the middle of this incredible run of form we played Antwerp in the UEFA Cup in mid-September. The lads were class over in Belgium. Peter Beardsley was at his dazzling best and Rob Lee got a hat-trick in the 5-0 win. Phillipe Albert was a recent signing and played that day. He was a good example of a Keegan signing: a great defender who could also play a bit. There was a real party atmosphere for the return match a fortnight later and we ran out 5-2 victors. This time Andrew Cole got a hat-trick. We were still unbeaten in the league when we played Bilbao at home in October. We started at an incredible pace and were 3-0 up after 20 minutes; however, they got two late goals and it ended 3-2; Kevin lost it about the crowd doing a Mexican wave after 20 minutes. We lost the away leg in a gut-wrenching 1-0 defeat to exit the cup on away goals. It didn't help that Andrew was out with shin splints.

Several key players were injured at this point, but at least we got Andrew's leg sorted with specialist help. There are several causes of shin splints, which is a generic term. As well as pain, he was also having some unusual symptoms such as numbness and pins and needles in his feet, as well as calf cramps. We took him to see an orthopaedic specialist in Leicester called Mike Allen. He inserted some pressure probes and diagnosed what we suspected: compartment syndrome. This is when pressure rises abnormally high inside a muscle. Muscles are covered in a thin sheet of connective tissue called fascia, which is very strong. When something causes the muscle to want to swell, it can do a little because of a protein called elastin bound to the collagen of the fascial sheath; this permits some stretch. Once the swelling reaches the limit of the elastin, the sheath can swell no more and this causes a steep rise in the pressure within the muscle, and the subsequent symptoms. Andrew had a very straightforward procedure to release the pressure and, to everyone's delight, it sorted out his issues almost immediately.

Towards the end of the year, Phillipe ruptured his ACL in training at Durham. It was a tough time for him. He was just starting in the team and they were having some great performances. He'd settled in really well. It's safe to say that Phillipe *loved* British culture, and especially Geordie culture. He immediately felt at home in the North East. He'd become a fan of *Viz* and did his best to learn the accent and dialect. He had his surgery and started the long road to recovery.

As a treat for the staff, we had a Christmas night out in Da Vinci's in Jesmond. Kevin and Terry were there with the coaches and physios. There was a lot of wine consumed that night. Towards the end of the meal, Kevin started to debate who was the faster runner, me or Faz. He can be a right wind-up-merchant when he wants to be so, of course, that started a heated debate. Terry had the bright idea of settling the dispute there and then, so we all spilled out on to the street. Terry and Kevin got us set up for a 50-yard sprint down Osborne Road. We waited for a gap in the traffic and were just about to go when a car suddenly pulled out from a side road. Realising that we were potentially sprinting into oblivion, we abandoned the race for the following day at training. Sure enough, Kevin and Terry, the comedy duo, hadn't forgotten, so Terry took bets on who would win, and we went out for the race. Terry set us away and, of course, I won. Kevin had his money on me, so he was over the moon. He was prancing about and decided that he wanted to give me a piggy-back. I duly obliged and Kevin ran about like a madman with me on his back for about 20 yards before collapsing in a heap. I thought no more of it until the next morning we heard Kevin wouldn't be coming in because he had a bad back. He needed a week off because he'd slipped a disc carrying me about! When he came back, he was literally bent out of shape for weeks afterwards. I hope he fined himself.

Then came a bombshell in early January: Kevin Keegan was selling Andrew Cole to Man Utd. It didn't make sense to a lot of people, knowing the advantage that would give Sir Alex's team. Once again, some fans were accusing the directors of 'selling the crown jewels'. Behind the scenes we suspected that too, because the club's infrastructure just didn't match the quality of the team on the pitch. Yet another overspend and clawback episode in Newcastle's history. To Kevin and Terry's credit, they famously went on to the steps at St James' and explained the difficult decision they had to make. The fans there at the time appreciated their candour and the moment was one that went down in the city's folklore. I do wonder how much the AWOL episode the season before had bugged Kevin. I think it had done enough for him to consider the pros and cons of a change up front. Paul Kitson was brought in. He was immediately compared to Andrew and the poor lad suffered a bit at the hands of some of the fans on occasion. Keith Gillespie came as part of the Cole swap deal but was received well by the fans, probably because they didn't see him as a like-for-like swap.

In February 1995 Kevin was asked to open a memorial to the 168 men and boys that died in the West Stanley pit disaster. He did that on Chester Road, beside the King's Head pub where I used to play football 20 years earlier. After that day we won four matches out of five, only losing to Liverpool away. But as so often happens here, disappointment slowly crept in while the season progressed after that purple patch, and from late March onwards our challenge for a UEFA Cup place the next season fell away and we finished sixth in the league. The spirits of the staff were lifted when we learned that the club was looking at a 300-acre piece of land for a new training ground at Woolsington. That was promising; a move towards a better environment for training and rehab would be significant progress in building a successful squad.

As we got into 1995, results picked up and offered promise, but we went out of the FA Cup in the quarter-finals to Everton. They're never a good team to lose to because there seems to be a bitter rivalry between both sets of fans for some reason. After that we had a patchy run-in. We won a couple, then only picked up two points from five matches. A big positive was that Phillipe was getting closer to returning to full training. One Sunday I was at Maiden Castle giving Lee Clark some treatment. Out of the blue, Phillipe arrived, followed shortly afterwards by Kevin Keegan. The manager was great with those one-to-one relationships. He'd told Phillipe that he would see him at the training ground to do some passing and controlling practice with the Belgian. Before long I heard Kevin effing and blinding in the changing room. 'Fucking Tommo,' he said. 'No fucking kit!' Ray Thompson worked as the sole kit manager at the time. He was lucky if he got one or two Sundays off a month. He'd left eight sets of kits out on the Friday afternoon before a match, in case there were any players coming in on the Sunday. Unknown to him, Faz had brought some of the reserves in on the Saturday morning for a session. They'd used all the kit. I heard Kevin call Tommo on the phone. 'Alright, pal?' he said. If Kevin called you pal, you knew you were in trouble. 'Where's the kit?' I heard Tommo trying to explain that he'd left a set of kits. 'Not here now, pal,' Kevin said as he cut off the conversation.

'Gaffer's radgie,' Nash said, laughing. 'Tommo's in trouble!'

We could hear Phillipe and Kevin talking next door. Every now and again one of them would come out with an expletive. Then we heard the familiar clack of studs on the floor and balls stotting off tiles, followed by the door slamming as they went out to the pitch. Then 40 minutes later Tommo burst through the door with a bag of kits. 'Where's the gaffer?' he asked.

'Ootside,' Nash answered. 'Tommo's in bovva!'

Ray jumped up on to the bench beside the wall and looked out of the narrow window at the top. He didn't say anything, then gave a little chuckle. 'Fucking hell.' He laughed again. 'I'm in trouble. Have ye seen the plight of those two?'

In a jiffy we were both up at the window. They must have raided the students' lost and found box for kit. Phillipe was wearing someone's dirty Durham Uni rugby kit, only two sizes too small: socks mid-calf, unbuttoned skin-tight rugby shorts and a top that just came to his bellybutton. Kevin had no socks on, skimpy yellow football shorts like something straight out of the early 80s … and a white vest just a bit too tight on the midriff.

'Bloody hell,' Nash said. 'That's one of England's greatest-ever captains out there.'

'Should I go out?' Tommo asked. He was shitting himself.

'No,' I said. They're nearly finished. There's no point. Tommo paced the floor for ten minutes, until we heard the door open, followed by the clatter of studs. Ray was out the room like a whippet out of the trap. 'Kevin, I'm sorr–'

'What you doin' here, Ray?'

'I brought clean kit.'

'No need for that, ye daft bugger!' Kevin said. He grabbed Ray in a playful headlock and rubbed his hair.

'Aye there was,' Ray replied.

'Don't be stupid.' So, Tommo had rescued the situation. Of course, he *had* done the right thing.

* * *

We managed to get a home win against Crystal Palace in the last match of the season, but we finished in sixth, one point behind Leeds. That meant we'd just missed out on a UEFA Cup place. Kevin was always positive and suggested the lack of distraction from Europe would aid next season's title bid. It was nice to see Blackburn win the title, though; my old Fulham mate Ray Harford was their assistant manager. We were all sad to see Derek Fazackerley leave, however. Ray managed to persuade him to return to Ewood Park and his native North West. Arthur took over as first-team coach. Faz was a great coach and a brilliant mate. It's hard to believe that he was only at the club for three years. There's no doubt his coaching legacy lived on during the remainder of the time that Kevin was at the club.

On the coaching side, Arthur had Steve Black to help him. Although Blackie was only part-time, he remained involved in the team's training methods (in 1995/96 he was also providing input to Sunderland who were in the First Division, and the rugby union club Newcastle Gosforth, who Sir John had just bought). He introduced a scientific approach to the players' performance. His mantra was that footballers only needed to be within 80–90 per cent of their peak fitness during the season. He said they weren't Olympians training for peak performance every year or so, but athletes required to win football matches for 40 weeks out of 52. His advice was that trying to get the players' fitness levels above 90 per cent would result in overtraining, fatigue and injury. His approach worked and we were blessed to have relatively few injuries in the years that he worked with us. He's remembered more now for his time in rugby, with the Falcons, Wales and the British Lions, but he was always expert in delivering sport-specific training to enhance skills and performance in whatever sport he coached.

During the close season, Ferra and I went to a sports medicine conference in Dallas for a week. It was Sir John Hall's idea. In many respects he was very progressive in his approach to sporting development in Newcastle. He brought a lot of ideas across from the States for the Metro Centre and he wanted to do so for sport as well. It was our first real experience of the US, and it was typical Texas, the most American of all the 50 states. The conference alone had 15,000 delegates. We were able to access different sports venues and events. We couldn't understand the attraction of baseball, and American football stopped too many times. Perhaps the most interesting from a professional perspective was a guided tour of the NFL's Dallas Cowboys training ground. It certainly gave us some perspective on how our facilities compared at the time.

Aside from sport, what truly amazed us was the amount of food there was. It was everywhere, and immediately available. Poor Ferra, we had so much to eat and drink while we were away, none of his clothes fitted him when the time came to go home, so he had to wear a pair of my jeans for the flight! His wife Geraldine didn't recognise him at first. She said he looked as if someone had taken a bicycle pump and blown him up.

Chapter 7

1995–1996

THE START of the 1995/96 season wasn't a good time for me personally. Things back home had been slowly going wrong. Having a husband who's a professional football physiotherapist takes its toll; we're just not there a lot of the time because of work commitments. To compensate for that I avoided socialising with friends inside or outside the club. That didn't work either and things came to a head; I separated from Lisa. Custody was awarded to her. I was allowed contact with Jonathan twice a week. That was a killer blow for me. All I could do at the time was push for more contact.

On the pitch, Kevin had transformed things. A team that usually comprised players from England and the rest of the British Isles and one or two 'foreigners' was slowly increasing the number of quality overseas players. He brought in new signings Les Ferdinand, David Ginola, Warren Barton and Shaka Hislop. David signed from Paris Saint-Germain (PSG). He was the perfect example of the class that was coming in from overseas, and eye candy for the ladies, too. With his quiet, gallic charm he went about his training sessions with athletic efficiency, giving us tantalising glimpses of the skills he was capable of.

It turned out we had a fortunate set of circumstances leading to him to coming to Newcastle. He was blamed for a last-minute error that resulted in France failing to qualify for the 1994 World Cup in the US and was being vilified at every ground in France. He wanted to get away from his country. Barcelona beat a group of top European clubs for his interest. Once they had his interest and intent, they took too long to seal the deal and several weeks elapsed. In stepped Terry Mac, who found David through his agent and called him. He told him how much Kevin and the chairman loved his style. He used his scouse charm to sell the city of Newcastle and, in no time at all, David had signed. What a coup by Tel!

Within a week of arriving, David was introduced to Geordie culture when Lee Clark and Steve Watson took him out for a couple of drinks and they ended up on a ten-hour bender. To be fair to the three of them, once they left the fume-filled changing room the following morning and were on the training pitch, you didn't notice. In fact, all three lads were very fit athletes. Les was no less impressive than them in training. He was great to have about the dressing room, with a great sense of humour and always taking the mick. On the pitch, something that impressed me about Les was his jumping ability. What a height he could jump to crash in some headers. He also had that knack of being able to hang in the air for that split second longer than a defender. Cristiano Ronaldo has that ability too. Les was just under six foot, but what he lacked in height he made up by leaping like a gazelle.

Playing football has a lot to do with the core muscles that anchor the pelvis and spine to the larger, ballistic muscles. The game itself involves a lot of starting and stopping, twisting and turning. If you can do those movements well, and also generate a lot of power that enables you to get off the ground quickly, perhaps to fire in a hard shot, then you have the athletic base that gives you a chance of being a great footballer. Of course, a footballer's brain is necessary as well. An aid to a great core is a low centre of gravity. That allows for great balance and explosive power from the area just above the pelvis. Les Ferdinand had all of that. Many taller centre-forwards, with notable exceptions, struggle with some aspects of the game other than heading a high ball. Being able to jump that extra 12 inches if you're of average height means you're still able to be the complete centre-forward, and that was Les. It helped that he was also hard as nails, with a presence about him on and off the pitch.

We started the season magnificently. The first match was at home to Coventry. The lads were wearing the beautiful and iconic shirts that summed up just about everything about the club: stripes, Brown Ale logo, blue star, Tyne Bridge, coat of arms with the seahorses and the old-fashioned buttoned-up collars as a shout-out to the past. Rob Lee scored early in the first half with a looping header, then Peter Beardsley sealed the win with a penalty in the last ten minutes. And didn't Les just look the part in the No. 9 shirt, scoring the third goal a minute after that. He'd been running around like a thoroughbred horse all match. Rob gave a great pass to him and he barrelled towards the Gallowgate End. Filan, the Coventry keeper, charged way outside his box, Les went past him down towards the right corner of the 18-yard area before banging the ball into the net; Terry Mac was jumping up and down like a jack-in-the box. It sounded like the roof lifted off for that Sir Les goal. He was the new No. 9 and the crowd was acknowledging that. He looked every part the gladiator they wanted him to be. Every player in the team that day was a class act.

The next match was three days later, down at Bolton. The lads were in the equally iconic maroon-and-blue away shirts that evening in Burnden Park. David Ginola ripped them apart. He was surrounded by quality up front: Peter Beardsley, Lee Clark, Rob Lee and battering-ram Les Ferdinand. Next we had an away win at Hillsborough. At the end of August, I sat at St James' when they hosted Boro, enthralled by the skill and relentless determination of the team: Peter, always class; Keith Gillespie, fast and accurate; Les, great target man; David, brilliant. Our 1-0 victory flattered our guests. Four wins out of four. We went top of the league. At the beginning of November we defeated a very impressive Liverpool team and by Christmas we were ten points clear of Man Utd. Towards the end of January we'd extended that lead to 12 points despite losing at Old Trafford in the Boxing Day fixture (on the 27th that year). It was at this time that Kevin strengthened the squad with Faustino Asprilla. The club was on fire, as was the city.

The whole region was buzzing. I'd been having a hard time dealing with my separation and not seeing Jonathan nearly enough, so Ferra had persuaded me to go out in Newcastle on a regular basis. At that time a lot of the players socialised in the Quayside area and we met up with them regularly. It became part of our lives. Meeting for a meal in Uno's with the players on a Monday evening became a regular fixture on our social calendar. The restaurant is situated beneath the beloved Tyne Bridge, possibly *the* most iconic symbol of Newcastle and its people. Of course, we usually had to do the obligatory pub crawl and visit a nightclub as well. It was such a wonderful time in hindsight; at every opportunity Ferra, Tommo and I met up with great guys like Lee Clark, Rob Lee and Steve Howey. The city was thriving too, emerging from the depression of the 70s post-industrial wasteland through the boom time of the late 80s. The Toon was gaining a reputation as a party city. People would come from all over the country for weekend breaks as well as drink-fuelled hen and stag parties. The success of the team percolated through to the psyche of the Geordies so the nights out were always great fun. On the whole, the players were professional in their attitudes and only went out when they were permitted. If they did otherwise, it would always get back to Kev via Terry Mac.

I started to gain more weight about this time. Kevin was always having a go at me about being overweight, so I accepted a £250 bet to lose a stone in three weeks. When I came in on the day of the weigh-in, I was still three pounds over. There were two runs at the Durham training ground, the river run and the forest run. Together they were about three and a half miles. I put on loads of layers and did both runs twice, as fast as I could. I was knackered but just scraped under the weight and won the bet.

After the turn of the year and with March approaching, many people in the city were starting to talk about winning the Premier League (or the FA Carling Premiership as it was called at the time). What could go wrong? Well, this club *is* Newcastle United. If it can go wrong, it will. It started to go wrong on 21 February 1996 when we lost 2-0 away to West Ham. Eleven days earlier we'd beaten Boro away, when Tino rescued the situation, coming on with just over 20 minutes to go and inspiring first a Steve Watson equaliser then a Les Ferdinand winner. Including the West Ham match at Upton Park, over a six-week period we played six times and dropped 14 points, including another six-pointer to Man Utd at home on 4 March. A week before that we witnessed a Keegan classic at Maine Road. The match ended 3-3 and Phillippe scored his second to get the equaliser in the last ten minutes. He nearly bagged a hat-trick that day, as Tino scored the second of our goals from a saved shot from the Belgian defender. Wouldn't that have been a collector's item: a centre-half hat-trick.

Then came the home match against Man Utd. We played brilliantly but Peter Schmeichel had one of those matches when, no matter what any of the lads did, we couldn't get the ball past him. Eric Cantona scored the only goal, one that ultimately sealed our fate and broke our hearts. All we knew at the time was that the stars had to align for the next nine weeks if we were to win the trophy. That match was David Batty's debut and the only home fixture we lost all season. But that anomaly belies what a great player Batts was. For the rest of the season what David did was to steady the ship. He became an anchor for the attacking players and broke down many a decent midfield opposition. He had great vision and awareness, nearly always hitting passes with precision. He had a work rate second to none. The funny thing about him is that he confessed to me that he didn't particularly like playing football. It was something he was very good at, so he did it to do his best for his family. He said the day he retired would be his last day in football and he has been true to his word.

Lee Clark missed out on much of the run-in because Kevin picked Batts before him. He always says we would have won the league if he'd stayed in the team. He certainly has a point. He'd been playing really well all season up to David's arrival. This is another of those frustrating 'what-ifs' from that season. Anyway, the last of this run of six matches dropping points was the 4-3 defeat away to Liverpool. That breathtaking match has been described as the best ever in the Premier League. For us it might have been so if we'd won. But the loss was soul-destroying. The lads played so well and the match lurched between hope and despair. Collymore's goal in stoppage time made me feel physically sick. It's without a doubt the worst feeling I had while at Newcastle United.

The element of doubt in our ability to win the league finally permeated through to the front of our minds. Why had we played so well and lost? Terry said later that he was sickened by the result, and Kevin said he was scarred. One thing was for sure, we now felt like the hunted, even though we were the ones who had to do the hunting for the rest of the season. Despite already surrendering our lead in the table to Man Utd, it was this match that introduced the real doubt that we could do it. The back-to-back defeats against Arsenal and then the Liverpool 4-3 were what finally made us realise we were mere mortals. Another significant blow was Steve Howey tearing his hamstring at Anfield, to add to an injury list that included Lee Clark and Keith Gillespie, putting pressure on Ferra and me.

An example of the pressure we were all under was John Beresford's substitution by Kevin in our 1-0 home win against Aston Villa. Bes was a top-drawer player as well as being a great lad. He totally deserved to be in that wonderful team but he fell foul of the gaffer that day. Kevin and Bes had already had a conversation beforehand about covering David Ginola. David drifted away at the start of the match, giving Villa a chance of scoring, so it was a 'told you so' moment for Bes and he vented his frustration and swore at the manager. You never did that sort of thing with Kevin, and Bes was immediately substituted. Robbie Elliott took his opportunity and remained in the left-back position for the rest of the season!

Kevin had his famous rant against Alex Ferguson on Sky Sports at the end of April. We'd just beaten Leeds away but the title was slipping away from us. The timing showed how much stress Kevin was under, because by then we were firmly the underdogs in the race, as the final results confirmed. That outburst from Kevin inspired the lads to try harder. That first week in May is one of my most painful memories in football. We'd managed three victories in a row, just about hanging on to Man Utd's coattails, praying they would slip up (they took 41 of a possible 45 points in their last 15 matches, and that broke us). We played Forest away; the tension was unbearable. Peter Beardsley put us ahead on the half-hour. He did what he was great at, lovely control, jinked past two defenders, then a third, and smashed the ball into the top left corner. We pressed them, Les hit the bar with a powerful header, only for an uncharacteristic mistake from David Batty to let Ian Woan through. He smashed the ball into the same spot that Peter had done about half an hour earlier. It was one of those head in hands moments. Many of our travelling supporters were in tears. One point really wasn't enough at that stage.

When it came to the final fixtures on 5 May, Man Utd were on 79 points and we were on 77, so we had to beat Spurs at home and hope Man Utd lost at Boro. If they drew, we could still be champions, but it was unlikely because they had a much better goal difference. We knew a victory over Spurs at home was well within our ability, but Boro beating Man Utd? That was real Hail Mary stuff. We clung to the hope that Middlesbrough were at home. As it happened, we drew with Spurs and Man Utd did what was expected of them at the Riverside, easily winning 3-0. Of course, Andrew Cole had to be on the scoresheet. We sat on the bench watching it all slip away. Well, listening really, because every time Man Utd scored 40 miles down the road we heard about it. It must have affected our players. I consoled myself by acknowledging it was too great a hurdle to cross. Nevertheless, the feeling of loss was awful. The fans were great when the lads went back out to do the lap of honour. They were, arguably, the greatest team to grace the cathedral that is St James' Park, but it was hard to take. Kevin tried to keep up a brave face, but his eyes betrayed the hurt inside.

I'd arranged to go for a pint with Ferra and Tommo at Rosie's Bar on the end of Stowell Street. None of us fancied it but we'd promised ourselves we would go out no matter what. Tommo had already gone down. Paul had finished off and was talking to my dad in the treatment room. I told them to go ahead. I would follow them down in 20 minutes, once I'd completed my tidy-up. Rob Gregory, the club orthopaedic surgeon, was still about so we left the ground together. There were still a lot of people milling around. Not far from Rosie's we noticed a bus swerve to miss something on the road. As we approached I saw two guys fighting. One of them had gone down and the other guy's elbow was pumping away … well, like a fiddler's elbow. I said to Rob, 'Bloody hell, that guy's taking a hammering … that's me dad!' He was the one on top doing the battering. We got closer and Dad walked towards us, followed by Ferra. I asked him what the hell was going on. He looked down at his hands. The knuckles on both hands were red and bleeding. 'What the … Dad! What were you fighting for?'

'He desorved it,' he answered. Ferra caught up, with a nervous smile and a shrug of his shoulders.

'Fuckin' hell, Derek; he's half-killed the fella!' he said.

'What happened?' I asked. He went on to explain. They were both walking down the hill, approaching Rosie's, minding their own business and chatting about the season. A man in his 30s shouted over to Ferra. He was the worse for wear on the beer already. He came over and gave Ferra abuse about being an Irish bastard and not understanding what missing out on the league title meant to the people of Newcastle. Ferra told him that of course he cared. He squared up to Ferra, so my dad had tried to stand in between them. He explained to the man that Ferra was as upset as anyone else about what had happened and that being Irish had nothing to do with it. Without warning the guy kicked my dad in the balls as hard as he could. Ferra said my dad just stood there for a second, staring. The other guy stared back. My dad then launched an attack on him. He went down in a flurry of blows. Dad kept up the punches as they both spilled on to the road. I think it was at this point that the bus and then my taxi swerved by. When he'd finished, the guy was unconscious. Ferra pulled my dad away. How on earth he sustained a kick to the testicles without going down like a bag of spanners I'll never know. After five minutes I went up the road to see how the guy was. Rob Gregory had checked him out and said he was okay; the paramedics were just loading him in the back of the ambulance. I could see that he was conscious and breathing, which was a big relief.

A few days later the police came to my parents' house in Gateshead and arrested my dad for GBH or something similar. They told him the man he'd 'assaulted' had a broken jaw and had required surgery. Dad was taken over to the police station on the corner of Pilgrim Street and Market Street and spent half the day there. He was interviewed by two detectives who said they were likely to have to charge him because he had no evidence to back up his claim that he was assaulted first and that he was simply defending himself. My dad said, 'What about this?' He lifted his shirt and loosened his belt. Across his lower abdomen was a bruise. He unbuckled the belt and dropped his trousers; down both legs, on the inside of his thighs from groin to knees, were two massive bruises. He said, 'I'll show you the state of my balls as well, if you want?' The detective said that wouldn't be necessary. They went off and had a chat. When they returned they said there was sufficient corroborating evidence to back up his story, so he was allowed to leave without being charged. As I said, I have no idea how he could take such an injury without collapsing to the ground. He was 57 at the time. If we were ever out in town with Warren Barton after that, he said my dad was his personal bodyguard.

Chapter 8

1996–1997

MY DAD had stopped walking like John Wayne by the start of the 1996/97 season. We didn't know it, but at the end of the previous season Kevin suggested to the board that perhaps he'd taken the club as far as they could go and offered to quit. The board were having none of that and offered him a very good contract and promised him enough money to get the job done. True to their word, they came up with £15m for the signing of Alan Shearer. I was away with the squad at the time, touring Thailand, Singapore and Japan. Ferra was involved in doing the medical back home.

Tommo and I knew something was up when Kevin left the queue for security at Manchester airport. He was standing beside Tommo when his phone went. He stepped aside to have the conversation, then spoke to Terry and left. We asked Terry on the plane who we were trying to sign. 'Italian left-back, that's all I can tell you, boys,' was as much as he would say. We forgot about it. The first place we went to was Bangkok. It must have been 95°F and 80 per cent humidity. Tommo and I had to load all the luggage into the back of a tiny truck. We were instantly lathered in sweat. There was no room on the bus so we had to climb into the back of the truck on top of the bags. That was our first introduction to

Asian traffic. The driver seemed to have a death wish. I'm not sure what was worse, the feeling of being slowly suffocated and cooked or that we were about to hurtle into the lorry in front of us that was doing emergency brakes every now and again for no apparent reason. When we got to the hotel, we were ready for a drink. The driver took one look at us and burst out laughing. 'Silk shirt, silk shirt,' he kept saying. He told us that the best thing for people like us was to wear a silk shirt. Peter Beardsley turned up to give us a hand unloading the bags. He did that whenever he could when we were away.

The first match was against the Thai national team, which we won 2-1. A lot of their supporters were wearing Newcastle shirts. Later that night we went out in Bangkok. Even back in the 90s that place was wild. Amid our wandering about the Royal City Avenue nightlife, often lost for words, we bought the silk shirts. We had a day to recover there before flying to Singapore.

The last match of the tour was against Gamba Osaka in Japan. We, the staff, promised ourselves a good send-off that evening. So, once we'd eaten at the hotel, Tommo and I put on our Bangkok silk shirts and went out to a few of the Keihanshin bars. We were flying home the following morning, which meant an early start for us to load everyone's bags into the truck. We got back about 2am and I set my alarm for 6am. At 7am my phone went off. 'Hello.'

'It's Peter.'

'Alright Peter.'

'Weren't you and Tommo loading the bags at six?'

'Aye. Why, what time is it?'

'It's seven. We're leaving in 15 minutes.'

'What?' For some reason my alarm hadn't gone off. I'm running about trying to get dressed and phoning Tommo at the same time. Tommo arrived downstairs at the same time as me. Peter was standing there with a big smile on his face. He's loaded all the bags himself then called us. What a star!

That Italian left-back Terry hinted at turned out to be Alan Shearer. He'd joined us in Singapore. Paul and I did our physios' assessment on him. His biomechanics weren't good at all. He was a bit flat-footed with a tendency to overpronate. He was an injury waiting to happen (that would be a chronic injury that could be career-ending). Up to that point in his career he'd never had an orthotic intervention for his biomechanics and gait. It's surprising how relatively minor problems with the anatomy of the foot and gait can affect the rest of the musculoskeletal system. Problems with the foot can result in hip and back issues, not to mention apparent isolated problems such as hamstring or calf strains. We had to decide: do we go for an intervention by correcting his arches with orthoses or leave things as they are? We discussed it with Alan and decided to not intervene, although we told him he was likely to have problems at some stage. I think what I said to Ferra was something along the lines of, 'He scores 30 goals a season with those feet, let's leave him alone!' Foot biomechanics sounds like a relatively insignificant problem, but it isn't really. Subtle correctional changes can sometimes have a massive effect, good or bad. That's why the services of an expert sports podiatrist are sought out by top clubs in the modern game.

When we returned to Newcastle we saw first-hand how Alan's signing had created a huge surge in emotion throughout the city, and many were already thinking, *Here we go again.* There was also the mouth-watering prospect of competing in the UEFA Cup. We came crashing down to earth when we lost the Charity Shield 4-0 to Man Utd. Despite that, we were still full of hope for the season's opener. After all, Kevin and Terry Mac were still there and our own Alan Shearer was back home at the top of his game.

We were desperate for a perfect start, but we lost two of our first three matches, only managing a home win against Wimbledon squeezed between a season opener away loss to Everton and a worrying home defeat to Sheffield Wednesday. Kevin then allayed our jitters when we went on a seven-match winning run, including away wins at Roker Park (the last away derby before they relocated) and White Hart Lane, as well as a breathless 4-3 home victory against Villa. Kevin had Tino, Les and Alan to choose from up front, with Peter just behind supplying them with ammo. All four of them were shining stars in another great team. The final match of that run was the famous 'Howay 5-0' rout of Man Utd at home. That meant a lot because of the 4-0 defeat in the Charity Shield, but more importantly the 1-0 defeat at home the previous season. Les said the irony was we played better in the match the season before and lost. I met one of my old schoolmates, Paul Tupman, afterwards. He'd always been a Man Utd supporter and he fully expected his team to win. The look on his face when I caught up with him was priceless.

What a phenomenon the combination of Ferdinand and Shearer was up front. Alan had all the attributes that Les had, including dominance in the air. He also had world-class finishing ability. His ratio of goals to chances was second to none. We were starting to believe again, nights out on the quayside were back on the agenda. Alan and Rob Lee became firm friends and they often accompanied Ferra, Tommo and me on evenings out. The people of Newcastle loved it. I think it's about that time that my nickname Del Boy stuck. Before Rob Lee introduced that moniker, if I did have a nickname it would be Wrighty or the Geordie version of Derek, Dekka. Rob had used it for a couple of seasons, but Alan picked up on it and used it until everyone called me Del Boy.

Looking back, it's such a pity that we never saw more of Alan and Les playing together than we did. After the victory over Man Utd, Alan needed surgery on his groin, meaning he was out for about four weeks from late October. Les then suffered a fractured cheekbone in the match against West Ham and was out for about six weeks. The Hammers match was a frustrating draw. They took the lead in the middle of the first half against the run of play, but then successfully defended until Peter finally managed to unlock their defence in the last ten minutes to make it 1-1. Les picked up his injury in a mad goalmouth scramble. Afterwards I took him to the RVI to have his face X-rayed. He was living in an apartment complex at the Newcastle racecourse at the time. Once we'd been sorted at the hospital, we went back to the racecourse to his flat. We went upstairs and he took me inside to meet his girlfriend in the living room. Dani Behr appeared. She was never off the television at the time. I knew who she was, but I had no idea she was his girlfriend. I looked at her, looked at him shocked, as if to say, *WTF, Les?* He laughed and gave me a wink. 'Derek, meet Dani. Dani … Derek.'

Fortunately, Alan returned from his surgery and took the centre-forward baton from Les while he was injured. The next match was away to Chelsea. It was towards the end of November. Al's return to play was successful and we got a draw at Stamford Bridge. However, he'd been having ongoing niggles with the other groin and Steve Howey had a couple of muscle tears that had taken a while to heal. Glenn Hoddle, the England manager, claimed to have had some success with the faith healer Eileen Drewery. Earlier in December, Kevin's wife Jean had recommended her good friend, Betty Shine, as a possible solution to some of our injuries. Betty was a medium and spiritual healer. Kevin packed Alan, Steve Howey and me off to Brighton to see her. Steve tells this story in a podcast, but there's a little bit more to the story than he tells.

The three of us were sceptical about faith-healing. I don't want to suggest it doesn't work, but on a personal level it implied to me at least that our professional ability as physios was being called into doubt. The two lads had their sessions with Betty, hopefully were healed, so we headed back to the hotel for the evening. A couple of the locals noticed the guys in the restaurant, had their photos taken, got autographs, etc. The lads were their usual gracious and accommodating selves. We went for a couple of drinks in the bar. By now word had got round that two England internationals were drinking in their hotel, so half the village came in to talk to us. It became an extraordinary night for them and developed into a drinking session. Eventually, we all took our leave and went to our rooms.

We didn't realise that the party went on for several hours downstairs and then some of the locals decided to find a room to sleep in. Several rooms were empty ... and unlocked, so they slept off their hangovers there. We thought nothing more of it until the day of the lads' Christmas party in December. It was fancy dress. We were going straight out after training at Maiden Castle and we'd hired a minibus to take us back in to Newcastle. Steve and I had got into our outfits, he was an emu and I was a fairy in a tutu. Alan wasn't yet in his fancy dress. Then all hell broke loose. Kevin's wife, Jean, had been on to Kevin during the training. Word had got back to her via Betty Shine that we'd all been involved in 'smashing up' a hotel down south. Apparently, Kevin was on the rampage. I was seeing to one of the players and could hear Kevin effing and blinding next door. Terry Mac came in and said he wanted to see the three of us. Alan went in and explained what had happened. We hoped it had done the trick because, when they came out, Kevin was having a laugh with him. Next, he brought Steve in. He seemed to be back in a bad mood. Steve, the bugger, sat down with the emu's head looking forlornly to the ground, but when he was talking he would move its head as if it was doing the talking. Kev then looked at me. 'Fuck's sakes, Derek,' he said. 'Look at the fucking state of you.' I just backed up what the others said, stood up and rearranged my tutu before picking up my wand and walking out with a skip in my step.

Kevin was having a laugh by this point. I went outside to catch up with the lads, putting on my pink Marie Antoinette wig. They were having a group photo. When they saw me a big roar went up. I tried my best to shush them but it was too late: Terry had jumped up on a bench in the changing rooms to peek through the window see what the commotion was. I saw his perm pop up first, followed by Ferra wearing a pirate's bandana and eyepatch. Then Kevin's face appeared. Tel and Ferra had big smiles on their faces while Kevin looked on in horror.

What Steve didn't mention in his podcast was what happened when we got back to Newcastle. The lads said we were starting in Rosie's bar, so the minibus stopped outside the Irish club and I got out, only for the driver to close the doors and drive off! Steve phoned me to say they were up at the ground, so I had to walk back up the hill in my fucking tutu and two-foot pink wig, wearing Doc Martens and carrying a wand. Bastards.

* * *

The good times can't last too long with the Toon, however. We didn't know, but the flotation of the club on the stock market was changing the dynamics between the board and Kevin. At the same time, over a seven-match stretch, we lost three and drew four. This run culminated in a loss away to Blackburn on Boxing Day. We know from Kevin's autobiography that he wanted to resign after that loss, but the board insisted he stay to see out the season, citing rules with regards to the transition to a plc. Football in England was going through its greatest transition. The old ways of mainly working-class supporters, many of whom chose to stand, watching First Division players who had no choice when they were bought or sold, were changing. The new corporate paradigm meant all-seater stadiums from 1994 (a legacy of the 1990 Taylor Report following the Hillsborough Inquiry) in the new Premier League, which started in 1992. Players had much more autonomy as a result of the Bosman ruling at the end of 1995. Most had agents by then. If a player was within six months of a contract expiry, he could arrange a pre-contract with a new club and leave on a free transfer. Add into the mix the huge amounts of money flowing into the game from 1992 onwards because of higher television payments from Sky Sports when they secured exclusive broadcasting rights, and it's easy to see now that this four-to-five-year period was the 'switch-flipping' period for the character of English football.

Newcastle United were at the heart of these changes. They'd just clawed their way out of the new First Division to get into the Premier League's second season. The Cameron Hall directors had taken control, the stadium had been redeveloped and a huge amount of money was coming to the club from television. The decision by Sir John Hall and Freddy Shepherd to float on the stock market as a plc meant the City also had to have a say. This was both from a financial perspective and a legal one because there were certain regulations that had to be followed. The board seemed to have their concentration elsewhere and Kevin found it difficult to even get in touch with any of them to discuss the situation.

More matches came up, we had two good wins over the remainder of the festive season. Next we went down to London for the traditional third round FA Cup tie at the turn of the year, to play Charlton. We drew 1-1 despite Kevin putting out his best team and Charlton being a division below. At least we hadn't lost, so the tie would come back to St James'. But then, three days later on 7 January, came the bombshell: Kevin Keegan had resigned. I hoped this would be another untruth, another baseless rumour, but time went by and he didn't return. I was shocked that he'd gone. Kevin's mood had darkened a little over the preceding months, but I put that down to the hangover of the previous season's disappointment. There was enough evidence that we'd turned the corner and that another 'Entertainers' season wasn't far away. The feeling of invincibility that Kevin instilled in the club had still been there.

The directors had summoned Kevin to a meeting at Sir John's house in Wynyard estate. A financier had been appointed as joint chief executive several months earlier to steer the club through the flotation. It must be said that the Cameron Hall directors were going to make millions of pounds from it. The financier was insisting that the gentleman's agreement Kevin had with the club to leave at the end of the season was not sufficient for a flotation and he had to either sign a new contract or leave immediately. The rest is history. By the time the story hit the news the following morning, Kevin was on the M25 with his family, heading for the Channel Tunnel and France. Kevin was manager at Newcastle for a five-year period between 1992 and 1997. When he started, 'old' football was ending in England. When he left, 'new' football had started.

Chapter 9

Kenny Dalglish

ONCE IT was obvious and officially confirmed that this time Kevin Keegan had definitely gone, some of the senior players were in tears. I was upset but tried to keep a brave face. I was also disappointed that I was unable to say goodbye to him and Jean. Over the years I got to know Jean well from functions or from her visits to the training ground and St James'. She loved the North East and I knew it would have been difficult for the whole family, not just Kevin. Terry took over on a temporary basis, assisted by Arthur Cox, until the club announced on 14 January that Kenny Daglish was to replace Kevin. Kenny was a good move by the board. The loss of Kevin was still an open wound, but the sentiment among most fans was 'at least it's Dalglish'. He certainly had the top-drawer player and manager pedigree that Terry's old Liverpool team-mate Kevin had. After all, he'd done the seemingly impossible in winning the Premiership with Blackburn Rovers only two years earlier. He would also be reuniting with the talisman of that campaign, Alan Shearer.

Kenny came out of retirement to take the job. Like a lot of men that I've met in football, Kenny was very different as a person to his TV persona. While being interviewed for television he often seemed to treat it as an adversarial encounter, but when I met him

I discovered he was warm and intelligent, and certainly not lacking the cutting humour that Glasgow is famous for. He undoubtedly had the same determination as Kevin to win. You don't get to the level of achievement that they both got to without it. Ferra and I got on great with him. Three working-class guys from three quite different parts of the UK that produced similar people. The club was in fourth place at the time of Keegan's departure.

To everyone's relief, Kenny kept Terry on. The transition was very smooth. It went from Kevin and Terry to Kenny and Terry. Dalglish was supportive from day one. He had that sense of humour but retained the ability to command respect without having to ask for it. One area where he was different to Kevin was discussing injuries with the press. Kevin tried to be as helpful as possible, giving details of the injuries with prognoses and timeframes. Kenny was the oppositive, being as vague as possible. In some ways that helped us. Terry continued to have an important influence in the dressing room as his assistant. He was always full of life and knew everything that was going on, loving a bit of gossip. He'd been Kenny's team-mate in the late 70s and early 80s, so why wouldn't Kenny keep him on? In football, you can't predict anything like that accurately, but Terry gave continuity with the Keegan era.

Kenny inherited a fabulous team that maintained its quality throughout the season. We were still in the UEFA Cup as well. Before the turn of the year we'd progressed through the first three rounds of the cup (Halmstads, Ferencváros and Metz) giving our fans some great European nights, both at home and away. Kenny's first UEFA Cup match in charge was a quarter-final tie against AS Monaco. We were without Les, Peter and Alan and were beaten by a rapid counter-attack when Thierry Henry got away and gave the ball to Sonny Anderson to score. So, the disappointment of a 1-0 home defeat.

Just before the Monaco away tie, Kenny took the team back to Anfield for a league match. There was a lot of talk about the 4-3 from the previous season. That was a one-off that would *never* happen again. We didn't start well and were three down before half-time. I sat there thinking, *Well this isn't going to be another 4-3.* At half-time, Kenny was having no negativity. He urged some respect and pride in the play. I think he couldn't face another three goals going in, especially with an important quarter-final coming up. The lads battled for everything in the second half and at least looked like coming away with some respect. Keith Gillespie scored with 20 minutes left, but after that the clock ticked down. At least we'd salvaged some pride. Out of nowhere we scored twice in the last five minutes to level the scores. The travelling Toon army were going crazy. Most remember the script: Robbie Fowler got their winner in injury time. Absolutely gut-wrenching and nauseating *again*. Another 4-3, and how bitter it was to take. Not quite as awful as the year before, though.

Then came the comprehensive defeat in Monaco. We had to deal with a lot of injuries at the time. For the away tie we had Tino and Peter back, but Alan and Les were still out injured. Alan was having a hard time dealing with the recurring groin injury. It was a great away day for the travelling Toon fans, but we struggled on the pitch trying to claw back the deficit against a Monaco team full of international stars, so it was a valiant effort, but we went down 3-0 on the night.

Nevertheless, in the league we remained in the top half of the table throughout the season. Over the course of the campaign, several members of the 'Entertainers' left the club, including Ginola to Tottenham Hotspur, and Beardsley to Bolton Wanderers. Kenny brought in Shay Given, Temuri Ketsbaia and Gary Speed, who were all popular signings. He also recruited Stuart Pearce, John

Barnes and Ian Rush, all of whom were in their mid to late 30s, and some supporters criticised him for doing so.

Off the pitch, there were some changes as well. Doctor Beveridge retired and we brought in our first full-time doctor, Roddy MacDonald. Roddy came from Celtic. He was a fully trained sports physician as well as a general practitioner. I also appreciated Ferra's contribution as a physiotherapist and we decided to share the on-pitch duties, which meant astute fans became aware that there were two of us. I certainly needed the help from Roddy and Ferra to shoulder some of the burden of injuries. The three of us would often go out socialising in Newcastle and would end up talking about our vision for the new 'medical department'. Speedo and Shay in particular became very good friends and were regulars on our nights out, usually with Alan and Rob. Shay was another Irishman who called me John Bull.

* * *

Towards the season's end we put in a good run. On the final day we needed to finish second for a European spot. We were the ones currently holding third, two points behind Liverpool. We also had to worry about Arsenal going past us if they scored more goals than us. It turned out to be a very different runners-up place to one year before. This time the lads were on fire, putting five past Forest at St James', which put Arsenal out of it. Meanwhile, down at Hillsborough, Liverpool had pulled back to 1-1 and Wednesday were down to ten men with an outfield player in goal. We thought the writing was on the wall. Seven minutes ticked by, but Liverpool couldn't score. That meant we qualified for the Champions League for the first time, as UEFA had just started to allow the runners-up of top European leagues to compete in the competition; more exotic travel for the fans. The results went the hardcore fans' way even more on the that final day because Boro and the Mackems were relegated as well. What a night in Newcastle that was, so different to the preceding season.

Chapter 10

1997–1998

IN THE close season, I was told that Newcastle were selling Les. This hit me hard. The combination of Alan and Les was unbeatable in my mind. Furthermore, Les was a great guy to have around the training ground and in the team. But, somewhere upstairs someone must have felt the need to balance the books. I'd heard rumours about it, so asked Les while we were on a run by the river at the Durham training ground. He told me he was gutted because he didn't want to leave Newcastle. The decision had been made and he had to live with it. What a loss. If ever a player deserved to be awarded the formal honorific address of 'Sir' as an informal accolade by the people as he was, it was Sir Les.

In the pre-season warm-up phase, we were playing in the Umbro Tournament involving Everton, Chelsea and Ajax. We were playing the Londoners at Goodison on Saturday, 27 July. The match was nearly over when Alan controlled a pass and went to lay it off, but then collapsed to the ground. I didn't see the mechanism of the injury, and his fall looked innocuous. However, he was obviously in distress. Other players were reacting as well, never a good sign. Alan had suffered a bad fracture dislocation that required to be immediately pulled into a better position. We knew straight away that he would be out for months. Times like these are always very difficult for players. They're bad for anyone, but for the players football is their passion and their livelihood. The club scrambled to try to stop Les leaving, but it was too late. We'd lost both of our star strikers for the start of the season, with the Champions League to compete in, too.

Years later, Les said he regretted leaving, saying he was too 'prideful' when Freddie Fletcher came back, cap in hand, as asked him to stay. He said if he had to make the decision again, he wouldn't have gone. I really wish he hadn't, too. We tend to forget that Sir Les was only at the Toon for two years. We also forget that the peak season of the 'Entertainers' was after Andrew Cole had gone and before Alan Shearer started. From our No. 9 perspective, that was the Les Ferdinand season. It was no surprise that he was named PFA Player of the Year for 1995/96.

We still had the best centre-forward in the country. Initially Alan was upbeat following his injury. In the first week or so he had the intense input as far as X-rays, scans and being reviewed by the orthopaedic surgeon. Our orthopaedic surgeon, Rob Gregory, was based in Dryburn Hospital in Durham. Rob was confident that we could get Alan back to full fitness; it would be some time, though. Once he had the surgery that was the difficult time for Alan. To start with he just had to rest. We were then able to get him in for some general cardiovascular exercises to maintain his fitness and muscle bulk. Working one side of the body has some effect in maintaining condition on the other side, so that's very important.

The real hard work started when Rob said Alan's leg could come out of the cast. Ferra had a good rapport with Alan so, although we shared the rehab, he spent most of his time with him while I coordinated the rehab of the other injured players. That seemed to work very well. I reverted to my old ways of working, with Ferra getting involved as well, as time would allow. But

Alan was a model patient and did everything asked of him by the programme we devised. Psychologically, he took a dip when he wasn't too far away from full fitness, but that's fairly common. It's often the hardest time for the professional athletes, trying to regain that final five per cent of fitness that sets them apart from 'normal' humans like the rest of us. This is when intensive effort is required. In the back of their minds, they're also wondering whether the injury is going to break down, or if they'll ever regain peak fitness.

Not to mention the pain. They often go through considerable pain at this stage. Joints are stiff, scar tissue has accumulated. The scar tissue must be broken down, often with painful deep friction massage from us, and the joint needs to regain its pre-injury range of motion. The stabilisers of the joint, as well as the ligaments, are the muscles and tendons, stimulated by the motor neurone nerves. The perfect functioning of the muscle-nerve interaction is something that we all take for granted but is actually complex. Fortunately, rehabilitating this mechanism requires only a little conscious thought from the athlete, but a lot of hard work. Simultaneous impulses must go to the tensing muscle and relaxing muscle while stretch receptors keep the reflex in check. Balance nerves in the joints also keep the brain aware of where everything is. All these nerves need to work in perfect harmony with the muscles to both protect the joint and produce the results in limb movements required – in Alan's case, wellyin' in a shot as hard and accurately as possible, while at the same time not ripping a muscle or spraining a ligament.

As Alan has admitted himself, after that second bad injury in his career (the first one was a ruptured ACL at Blackburn), he was not back to 100 per cent for that explosive initial movement that benefits a top-class footballer. That's where our experience and knowledge came in. We were able to work on Al's balance nerves, while helping him to recruit as many motor units as possible to work the muscles in a strong, coordinated way. We then had to reassure him that he was doing fine.

* * *

We were short on forwards. Huge stars such as Les, David Ginola and Peter Beardsley had left the club. Kenny had brought in Jon Dahl Tomasson but had turned to Tino as his first-choice striker. In the opening Champions League group stage match, Wednesday, 17 September, we recorded a famous victory over Barcelona. The greatest referee in the word, Pierluigi Collina, with his staring eyes and shaven head, was in charge that night. Keith Gillespie had an amazing match. What a blessing to be so fast and skilful that you can sail past one of the best defenders in the world and deliver inch-perfect crosses. He said later it was his greatest performance. Tino scored a hat-trick, one of the most memorable nights in our history. His second and third goals were headers courtesy of Keith's crosses, when the Colombian made them inch-perfect by leaping like a salmon out of the Tyne. He then capped it off with his effortless slow-motion handspring in celebration.

In October the lads had an away tie in Kyiv. We'd experienced problems with players coming down with diarrhoea and vomiting bugs while travelling abroad, and Ukraine had recently gone through a split from the Soviet Union, so the directors decided we needed to take with us all food and drinks required by the players. This was a significant logistics endeavour and Tommo was left with the responsibility of sorting out getting the supplies, which had been brought from the plane, from the lorry. He needed a hand, so the two of us spent an hour or so humping all the food – steaks, salmon, etc., plus bottled water – into the kitchen. Tommo gave two security guards US$30 each plus bars of chocolate for each of their children to guarantee they made sure none of the food went missing.

We were sharing the same room, five storeys up. No lifts. We found our bags and carried them up the stairs. The rooms were just as you would expect for a country recently emerged from the grip of the Soviet Union: lights not working, sockets hanging off the wall. Ray went to look out of the window. 'Derek, Derek,' he hissed urgently. 'Come and see!' One of the security guards was running to a waiting car carrying two bags of salmon. 'Shite, Derek, there's ganna be nee food left.' As the guard was returning from the car, I banged on the window. He looked up and we both waved. I pointed to my eye in the universal language that says 'seen you'. We waved again. He slowed his jog to a walk and gave a sheepish wave back. At least we had enough food to last the trip. I must say that when we made the same trip in September 2002 they'd made remarkable progress once the restraints had been taken off their country.

On the evening before an away match in Europe we usually went to the ground for a training session. Prior to that I would set up a treatment room in the hotel. I meticulously laid out the tapes and bandages with the other kit so the lads who required it could have whatever they needed applied. If any needed a massage, the masseur, Mick Greener, helped by Len Clarke or John Huntley, would be there as well. So, in Kyiv, between 5.30pm and 6.30pm the preparations for training would be done, we would leave shortly after that and start training about 7pm. But I was unable to do any of the preparations at the hotel for the Kyiv match because of humping boxes of salmon and steaks and befriending their security guards. So I was running round at the ground like a blue-arsed fly, applying tapes and strapping as quickly as I could. I was lathered in sweat, stinking of salmon and blood from the steaks.

Kenny started his pre-season talk: 'Lads, just before I get started … Derek, in future could you sort all the taping and strapping at the hotel before we get here? Thanks.' Terry's standing beside him, nodding and rubbing his chin wisely. I looked at Tommo, who had a big grin on his face. The players who knew what I'd been doing were having a giggle too.

'Aye, Gaffa, no problem.'

The following evening the lads fought for a good 2-2 draw, coming back from two goals down. When we got back to training at Darsley Park I had a word with Kenny. Not long after that, Tommo got an assistant! George Ramshaw was another addition to our staff, and what a great guy he was to have around.

In the Champions League the glory still wasn't to be, as we eventually finished third in the group behind Dynamo Kyiv and PSV Eindhoven. Two back-to-back defeats against PSV were what did us in, meaning even if we beat Kyiv at home in the final match we couldn't go through. The two goalscorers for us in that dead-rubber match against Kyiv were John Barnes and Stuart Pearce. John Barnes used some neat skill to beat a defender and fired home after a surging run through midfield by David Batty, then Stuart hit a sweet 20-yard 'psycho-style' free kick into the top left corner. We'd won 2-0 but failed to progress.

John and Stuart had become good friends by then. Barnsey was a lovely guy. He was bright as a button and always wanting to engage in conversation. Every morning we would be greeted by him with questions about what we'd been up to the night before. That could lead the conversation in any direction. He had a tremendous general knowledge and sought out discussions. He always respected our opinions and was genuinely interested in lively debate. Yes, John was one of my favourites. On the pitch, his legs were starting to go a bit but he was still the best passer of the ball I ever saw play for Newcastle. He always hit his man, never gave the ball away and I never saw an opponent ever cut out a pass.

Stuart was another of my age contemporaries, like John. We had a love for punk rock; we were both teenagers in 1977 when punk was massive in Britain, although Stuart is really a punk rock super-fan. We went to see bands together when they came to Newcastle. The Cluny in Ouseburn was a great spot, and we saw the Stranglers and Stiff Little Fingers there. Stuart was also a thinker, despite his psycho reputation. He had a very astute analysis of matches. Despite his ability to think tactically he was mentally strong and, yes, was hard as nails, both from the perspective of being willing to mix it with anybody but also extremely determined. I always thought if I'd made it as a player, that's how I would want to be.

Evidence of his mental toughness was his response to a lingering hamstring injury. This was at the time we were starting to use MRI scans more and more, but the quality of the scans wasn't like today, and the grading scales for injuries weren't to the modern standard. He had a T-junction injury to the biceps femoris, but the scan was falsely reassuring. I wasn't so sure from a clinical perspective, but we decided to rehab Stuart according to the scan. We'd progressed carefully through the rehab but he broke down when just about ready to return. That meant we had to go back to square one, starting all over again. Not only that, but we had to take much more time and care because we now knew the original injury was more severe (as was suggested clinically). That was a lesson for me and Ferra, but Stuart had to accept that he was out for more weeks. He never complained and never moaned once, just got straight back to it and worked back to full fitness like the professional he was.

Come 1998 we were struggling in the league and out of Europe. Tino Asprilla left to re-join Parma. Sir John also stepped down and Freddy Shepherd took over as chairman. Things were starting to look a bit shaky; the fans were getting restless. Alan was still out injured, and we desperately needed him back. He was making tremendous progress, though. He returned for his first match back as a substitute at home to Bolton on 17 January – that's only six months out. Ferra and I sweated out that match, but he came through fine. We were all proud of that achievement.

It was a very different team that he was coming back in to, though. He did well in that match, but our experience with the professionals coming back after a significant injury was usually not problems with the first outing, but the second and third. The first match they would usually get through on the buzz of adrenaline and often a short period on the pitch. No matter how hard the fitness coaches work with the players, they really don't have full fitness unless they're playing. When a returning player then gets a 90-minute run-out on their second or third appearance, they can really struggle and are at risk of picking up another unrelated injury. Fortunately, that wasn't the case with Alan. He thought he'd lost a yard of pace, but they often feel that for the first half a dozen matches or so.

At the beginning of March, Kenny arranged a bonding trip to Ireland for the first team, but didn't travel, leaving Terry Mac in charge ... That was when the infamous 'incident' in a Dublin pub happened between Alan and Keith Gillespie. Tommo and I were there for the start of the drinking session but weren't there at the time of the 'battle'. Terry had arranged for us all to have a meal at the hotel at 7pm. We as non-player staff *had* to be there on time, so we made our goodbyes and reminded the players that they would have to follow shortly after. Unlike the players, if we failed to turn up, we might lose our jobs, so even though it was tempting to stay and party, it wasn't worth it.

I remember Alan saying, 'Aye, aye, Del. See ye later.' He had that look on his face that said he had no intention of following us. We left, got back to the hotel and showered. We joined Terry and a couple of staff in the restaurant. Seven o'clock came and went. Terry started to get agitated. He asked us where they were, so we told him: Café en Seine. He made a couple of phone calls and calmed down. 'It's okay lads, they're on their way back now,' he said.

Meanwhile, back at the pub, the drinking intensified, and they'd started a drinking game. Alan's another wind-up merchant, and during the game he managed to upset Keith, who was not much of a drinker and consequently was losing each round. Alan said something and Keith suggested they took it outside. Never one to back down, Alan took it outside. Keith tried a sneaky pre-emptive swing but missed and the England captain hit him once and he collapsed to the floor, smashing his head on a plant pot. Keith lay there motionless. Alan thought he'd killed him. To everyone's relief, Keith was still breathing, even though Steve Howey couldn't get him to wake up. An ambulance was called and Steve jumped in the back with him. Keith spent a night in one of Dublin's hospitals.

The news eventually filtered back to Terry, who was beside himself. The lads started to arrive back at the hotel, worse for wear. We managed to calm Tel down. The following morning, Ferra and I went to the hospital to see Keith. We took some fresh clothes for him. The press by this stage had started to gather at the front of the hotel. Keith was fine, other than having a terrible headache. He had no recollection of the events whatsoever. He stayed in the hospital until it was time to go to the airport, and one of the staff took him straight there to avoid the press.

It didn't end there. Keith had gone home early to avoid the press. The following day the lads were out again. For some reason Stuart Pearce took a liking to a traffic cone. He spent most of the afternoon with it on his head. Somehow the traffic cone ended up smashing a lady's car window. At least Stuart left her a note and a cheque to cover the damage.

Then, on 15 March came the *News of the World* sting, when investigative reporter, Mazher Mahmood, secretly recorded Freddy Shepherd and Douglas Hall in Marbella criticising the fans and the people of Newcastle in general. The backlash was so intense, causing ten days of chaos and turmoil at the club; they both had to step down and Sir John returned as chairman. Sir John had really had enough of running the club. It wasn't something he'd ever wanted to do, but he took it on for the second time because he was the only man for the job.

* * *

After a poor run of form in the league we finished 13th. Dalglish's style of football was inevitably compared to Keegan's; it was considered by many to be 'unentertaining', making Kenny's management unpopular with some. Despite a disappointing position in the league, we reached the FA Cup Final by beating Sheffield United 1-0 at Old Trafford, when Alan scored on the hour. A great day out for the fans in London beckoned. The final was against Premier League winners Arsenal on 16 May. They were looking to win the double. A trip to London for the FA Cup is always a great weekend for the Toon fans, but the final itself was an anticlimax; we never really threatened to win, going down 2-0. As the Gunners had won the double, Newcastle's silver lining was qualification for the last-ever European Cup Winners' Cup. Perhaps that helped justify the open bus tour when thousands turned out in the city, despite us losing the final. It was an amazing and unexpected response from the folk of Newcastle, but it was a bizarre experience for us because we hadn't won anything.

Chapter 11

Ruud Gullit

IN THE close season, Freddy Shepherd reinstated himself as chairman and Douglas Hall returned as a director. Kenny signed Didi Hamann, Nobby Solano and Laurent Charvet. After just two draws at the start of the 1998/99 season, he was sacked by Freddy, being replaced the same day by Ruud Gullit. That was one of the most unexpected managerial changes in my time at the club. We were only two matches into the season and the previous result was a 1-1 draw away to Chelsea. Shepherd said Kenny had offered to resign at the end of the previous season, but the departing manager denied this. Kenny claimed the first he knew about it was through the press. He later went on to say that nothing, including the cities of Glasgow and Liverpool, compare to Newcastle for the obsession and devotion to just one club. I was shocked and saddened by his departure. He always looked out for his staff and we really appreciated the continuity we had with Terry staying on after Kevin went. When Kenny went, Terry went, so that was a double loss to us. We also lost Steve Black as well. He'd been head-hunted by Graham Henry, the new Wales national rugby union team head coach.

Ruud was a huge appointment, having played the game so well at the highest level. He'd also started his managerial career successfully, winning the FA Cup with Chelsea and getting them to sixth in the league. The following season he'd been sacked with no clear reason offered by the club. Ruud had been out of management for about six months when we appointed him. The rumour among the Newcastle staff was that at Chelsea it was his assistant Graham Rix who did all the heavy lifting and was the main reason for their success. When I first met Ruud, he was very charming; he assured us all about our roles being safe. He brought in Steve Clarke as his coach. He also tried to change certain aspects of the players' culture and tried to improve the food the lads were eating after training. It was more of a Mediterranean diet style.

Our first match under Ruud was Liverpool at home. They hammered us. Michael Owen scored a hat-trick. He rubbed his hands together in glee when he scored his third. I'll never forget that. The press suggested he might have had a bet on scoring a hat-trick, but most Geordies saw it as excessive pleasure at scoring against us. We lost the next match away to Villa. One of the first things Ruud did was to promote John Carver to be an assistant coach for the first team, alongside Steve Clarke.

At that time the future should have been promising again, with some great professionals at the club: John Barnes, Gary Speed, Stuart Pearce, Batts, Rob, Shay, Alan. It wasn't long before the same pros started to report that things were not well with them: sentiments like, 'Gullit's arrogant', 'Doesn't like Alan at all', 'Thinks Al has too much power'. The players were all supportive of Alan. From my perspective, I never formed much of a relationship with Ruud. It wasn't his style to engage with the physiotherapy staff. Fair enough, all managers have their own styles. He left day-to-day discussions about injuries to his coach Steve, who was great.

Ruud banished Rob Lee, Stuart Pearce and John Barnes to train with the reserves and it didn't take him long to sell David

Batty to Leeds. A famous moment came in training when he told Steve Howey to force Alan on to his left side because he 'has no left foot'. That was in earshot of hundreds of watching supporters … and Alan. Things continued to deteriorate. Ferra was convinced he was going to lose his job. The thought crossed my mind for me, too. It didn't help that we were overworked, with little of the finance coming from television to the club trickling down to the medical department.

We picked up three good wins in September, but in October were knocked out of the Cup Winners' Cup in the first round. We'd beaten Partizan Belgrade at home but lost away and went out on the away-goals rule. Not long after going out of Europe, Ruud sold Steve Watson to Aston Villa. Yet another one of the Geordie old guard was gone. What a servant the North Shields lad had been to the club. He was with us for seven years and played in positions all over the pitch. He was the model professional, always putting everything into training and matches. He was always super-fit, capable of keeping up his work rate to the final whistle. He was a big miss for the squad.

We moved to training at the Durham County Cricket Club's ground at the Riverside in Chester-le-Street. The internecine struggle continued. That was when Ferra suggested Ruud might have the dressing room bugged. So, we did a search of the room, including looking in the roof space. We didn't find any recording devices! On the positive side, Shola Ameobi emerged from the youth team to establish himself in the first team and, in November, Gullit brought in big Duncan Ferguson from Everton, we thought probably as a replacement for Alan. Dunc and Alan immediately became firm friends.

Ferra's dad died. My friend had always been very close to his family back home in Northern Ireland and it was a tough time for him. When he returned he was left with an even greater impression that his days were numbered. With the state of things at the club it was an upsetting time. Ferra and John Carver were good mates but they'd been pitted against each other in the struggle. Kevin had only been gone a couple of years, but how things had changed from those carefree mornings at Maiden Castle.

A pleasant relief from the struggles came in November of that season. England were playing Scotland up at Hampden Park in the first leg of the Euro 2000 qualifiers. Alan was playing for England. Kevin was now England manager. How the hell did that happen so soon? We were able to get tickets and met with some ex-Scotland players, including Darren Jackson and Stuart McCall, before the match. My brother was working as an A&E doctor in Glasgow at the time and he came along.

England put in a solid professional display. To open the scoring, Scholes chested down a through ball from big Sol Campbell and put it away, then he headed in a Beckham free kick just before half-time. Great day out and we won 2-0. Straight after, we went to Lanigan's Bar in Shawlands Cross, just up the hill from Hampden. The pub was packed with Scotland supporters drowning their sorrows. There were a handful of England supporters with us, hiding our flags and keeping quiet. Ally McCoist was there. My brother had met him before, through Barry Venison. He was chatting to Ally and asked if he would sign his England flag. He produced a tiny corner of it and Ally signed. Standing beside Ally was Derek McInnes, who was playing for Rangers at the time. Derek signed as well.

Standing in the bar next door, holding court, was the Rangers and Scotland (and Sunderland) legend, Jim Baxter. Ally McCoist had the bright idea of getting Jim to sign the flag as well. Jim was more than happy to sign it. In fact, he was so keen to sign it, he whipped it out of my brother's coat pocket and waved it around. 'Be proud of your flag, son,' he shouted. Well, there's pride and there's stupidity. He then proceeded to announce to the 50 or so Scotland supporters that he was signing a St George's Cross. I looked into the bar thinking, *Here we fuckin' go*. It was obviously a Rangers pub, and Jim knew that; I swear in that moment you could tell exactly which ones were the Rangers supporters (most of them, fortunately) and which ones weren't. There were one or two very pissed-off looking faces, but when a cheer went up for Jim Baxter, I knew we'd be okay. My brother gave me the flag. I wish I knew where it is now.

Then came the FA Cup semi-final, Toon against Spurs at Old Trafford. Les Ferdinand and David Ginola were playing for Spurs. It was rumoured that Spurs hadn't sold their tickets and there were Geordies sitting among some of their supporters. It was such a draining match for the lads, end-to-end for 90 minutes. It went to extra time. Didi Hamann and Speedo linked up so well with Alan and Duncan. Andy Griffin ran his heart out. Shay was his usual calming influence in goal. Spurs had enough chances to win but didn't take them. From nowhere, Sol Campbell handled the ball in the box. Big Duncan even remonstrated with the ref when he blew the whistle because he thought he'd given Spurs a free kick, but it was a penalty for us. Alan took it. Ruud was sucking on his gold pendant, but his centre-forward assuredly put away the penalty. The icing on the cake was Al's second goal, a screamer hit with the outside of his foot into the top corner; one of his best.

In the final against Man Utd at Wembley, the fans as usual took over London for the weekend; peaceful Trafalgar Square infestation by the black-and-white hordes has become a Geordie tradition. The night before the final, Ruud summoned Ray

Thompson. He told Tommo that he wanted him to go into the kit room and lay out the players' boots in a 4-4-2 formation with Harps in goal. For Tommo to choose the correct boots, Ruud showed him the starting XI for the following afternoon. He was sworn to secrecy. At one o'clock in the morning he had to return to the room and place the boots back where they needed to be. To this day he swears he has no idea why he had to do it. Ruud also asked him sprinkle salt across the dressing room floor at Wembley before everyone else arrived. We presumed it was to bring grace and ward off evil spirits. Tommo said he couldn't bring himself to do it. Ruud checked and, because it hadn't been done, he did it himself. Ferra told me blessed salt was a Catholic tradition.

Despite the sacramental, the match ended in another massive disappointment. The lads tried their hardest, but on the day the team didn't perform. Ruud had decided to go with Harps in goal. United scored after 11 minutes through Teddy Sheringham, with Andrew Cole involved in the build-up. Paul Scholes scored early in the second half to take the wind out of our sails. We lost 2-0. What a nightmare, two FA Cup Final defeats in a row. That meant another open-top bus tour of the city. It's very humbling and amazing how many people turned out for these two tours despite us not winning anything. The lads didn't really want to do the first one, and they hated doing the second one, not because they didn't feel a strong connection with the supporters, but because they'd failed and were embarrassed. Like the preceding year, tens of thousands of supporters came on to the streets to cheer us. They climbed up lampposts, hung out of windows, stood on roofs, waving their black-and-white flags and scarves.

At one particularly busy intersection, the bus PA system was playing 'Blaydon Races'. Ruud turned to me and said, 'What's this fucking shit music they're playing?'

'It's the Geordie national anthem, Ruud: "The Blaydon Races".'
He didn't hear me because the noise of the supporters singing it was
too loud. At least playing in the final meant we qualified for the
UEFA Cup, despite finishing a disappointing 13th in the league,
the same position as the year before.

* * *

Before the season started, the doc Roddy MacDonald told me he
was leaving. As well as being a great sports physician, Roddy was a
good mate so that was news I didn't want to hear. Kenny Dalglish
had been appointed as director of football at Celtic. He and John
Barnes, the new head coach, had asked Roddy to join them as the
doctor. That was an offer he couldn't refuse, so he was off. When
pre-season training got underway we started doing trips to play
some away matches. The first of these were three matches in three
days in the Netherlands. We were based in Eindhoven. When we
arrived at the hotel, most of the young fans chasing autographs
crowded around Alan. One or two went to Ruud first. He looked
genuinely surprised that Alan was so popular. He told all the
players that the first night there was a free night. We thought it
was a test. If it was, the British players failed it: they went out on
the lash. I think one or two of our group had their 'cards marked'
by Ruud after that. Just to add to the list.

A couple of days after returning from Eindhoven we were
playing at Tannadice against Dundee United on Thursday, 22
July. Steve Clarke told me he had to speak to me about something.
Here we go, I thought, *it's time to move on*. He asked me, on behalf
of Ruud, to distance myself from Ferra. There was now a clear
division within the club between Ruud and some staff and some
senior players. Ferra was very close to Alan following his fracture
rehab and was therefore considered to be very much on Alan's side.

It all seems very childish in hindsight, but sometimes football can be like that. At times close bonds can result in meteoric rises in the sport. Other times it gets you sacked. There's often no rhyme nor reason to it. It's simply human nature (*masculine* human nature). My way of dealing with this throughout my career was to try to get on as best I could with everyone without making a public song-and-dance about any friendship I had. At that time, however, I had to make an immediate decision. It was a no-brainer. Steve was in a difficult situation but I told him my friendship with Paul was too strong to break because of a perceived feud between the boss and his senior players. There was nothing pleasant about the situation I was putting myself in at all, but I was having nothing to do with taking sides. At least I would sleep easy at night, even if I lost my job.

Two days later we were down south playing against Reading, and I saw another aspect of Ruud. He put himself on the team sheet as sub. He came on at the start of the second half. What a player! On the pitch the man is a colossus. It was as if he had a ten-yard hemisphere of influence around him. He won everything near him, in the air or on the ground, then hit his man without effort, spraying accurate passes here, there and everywhere. It was one of these passes, a long ball to Paul Robinson, that got us a penalty and subsequent goal.

Prior to the start of the new season, Ruud brought in Marcelino after he'd done well for Mallorca the season before. He also brought in Kieron Dyer from Ipswich and sold Stuart Pearce to West Ham. Ruud never gave Stuart a chance at Newcastle. He went on to play two seasons for the Hammers in the top flight, then captained Kevin Keegan's Man City to the First Division championship. For a while before he left Stuart had nowhere to stay because he had a good idea he was being sold and the lease on his house was up. He ended up sleeping in my flat in Chester-le-Street for three weeks. I had my son, Jonathan every other weekend. Stuart slept in Jonathan's bunk bed when he was at his mam's, but when he was with me Stuart was relegated to sleeping on the settee. Then the move to London came through and he was gone.

The last pre-season match was in Germany, against Bochum. Alan scored two, but we lost 3-2. While we were away, Tommo told Ruud that he needed the final players' list to submit to the EFL (English Football League) before the start of the season. Ruud said he would speak to him at the airport. While we were waiting for the flight, Ruud took Tommo to a quiet spot and went through the squad and their numbers. Rob Lee was missing from the list. Tommo pointed that out to Ruud. The manager said he wasn't getting a number. Once again he was sworn to secrecy. As soon as we arrived back in Newcastle we all went straight to the Quay Club on Dean Street. Most of the players were already in. I followed Tommo down the stairs. At the bottom I spotted Rob Lee (who hadn't travelled) leaning against the wall with a bottle of beer in his hand. 'Thompson, you're a fucking wanker,' he shouted.

'What?' Tommo replied.

'Fucking *Sunday Sun* just phoned me, innit.'

'What ya talkin' aboot, Rob?' Tommo asked. Rob proceeded to tell him that the papers already knew that he hadn't been given a squad number. Less than five hours after Ruud had told him and he was sworn to secrecy, someone had already called the papers and told them!

* * *

We lost the first three matches of the 1999/2000 season, then managed a draw at home to Wimbledon. Even in that match we'd given away a 3-1 lead. We started to hear the mutterings of discontent about the manager from some supporters. Internally, the atmosphere was probably the worst I can remember. To be fair to Ruud, his only English signing, Kieron Dyer, had made a promising start. Alan nicknamed him 'Pinhead', and that was shortened to 'Pin'. Ruud had told Kieron that he didn't like British players because they drank too much alcohol, but he'd done his homework on him and he didn't fit into that mould. We were amused by that because Pin certainly liked his nights out with the lads on the quayside.

Then came what was to become one of the biggest matches in the club's modern history: Sunderland at home. It was the fifth match of the season and we had only one point. By now the whole city knew there was a feud, but no one expected what happened next: Ruud dropped Alan and Duncs for the match. Duncan's popularity wasn't far behind Alan's. The staff had an idea that it was happening because in preparation Ruud had Alan and Duncan playing for the reserve team against the first team. He spoke to Ferra, telling him it was 'the dawn of a new era at St James''. Ferra told me he was expecting his P45 at any time. Ruud didn't speak to the two forwards to tell them that they weren't playing; it was up on the team sheet for them to see, though.

It was a summer's evening match, played towards the end of August. It became unforgettable. The heavens opened; floodlights were needed because it was so dark. Half the ground was still uncovered, and thousands were soaked to the skin in the pouring rain. I walked down the tunnel with Tommo, and we passed under the 'Howay the Lads' sign. Ray looked at me and shook his head. The club was tearing itself apart at team level. The outcome of this match was more than three points and bragging rights over our rivals. When play started an almighty roar went up into the black sky and bounced back from the bank of clouds into the cauldron. No flares required here tonight. Kieron grabbed the first goal and we went in 1-0 up at half-time. When the second half came, the punishing rain intensified. It was coming down in silver sheets. Spirals of rain swirled around in the lights before streaming down on to the players. The supporters were so wet that some went bare-chested. Clouds of steam lifted off the terraces. Big Duncs came on as substitute to rapturous applause from the Toon army, who were now slightly delirious in the monsoon conditions.

Most of us sitting on the bench (and in the crowd) sensed something bigger than the match was happening. That night the rain was the emotional turmoil going through the club and city. Only, when we were 1-0 up, the score and the conditions didn't align. But then, just over an hour in, Niall Quinn rose and headed the equaliser in front of the Leazes End; it was starting to align. Alan was brought on, but straightaway Kevin Philips put Sunderland ahead. Alan must have known in the last 15 minutes he could have saved Gullit's position. If the thought did cross his mind, it would never have stopped him from scoring if he could, he was too much of a professional ... and a Newcastle supporter for that. It wasn't to be, we lost at home to the Mackems. One point from five matches. I've never experienced a match like that before or since. I felt in my heart something was about to happen sometime in the next week or so. The stormy Wednesday defeat to the local rivals told us that.

I was usually the first member of staff at the training ground. It was rare to see a player in before me. The following morning I was pottering in and about the physios' room when I spotted Duncan heading for Ruud's office. Not long after I saw Alan. It was clear from the looks on their faces that they were still blazing angry. I decided to leave them to it. They both took a turn in telling Ruud what they thought of him. I would have loved to have been a fly on the wall for that!

After the Sunderland fiasco there was a lot of unhappiness among the fans. No matter how big a footballer he'd been or how well he'd done as a manager at Chelsea, Ruud would never come close to Alan, or even Duncan, in the eyes of the supporters. Freddy Shepherd had a reputation and track record for abrupt sackings, but at the Thursday press conference Ruud did himself no favours by blaming Alan and Duncan. He implied that the team's loss stemmed *from* the substitutions. That should have been enough for him to go, but what also did for him was that before the match he said the Milan derby was more important than the Newcastle-Sunderland derby. A lot of English football supporters might agree with him, but none of them are from the North East.

Ruud broke the tension when he resigned on the Friday morning. Relief was the main emotion I felt. I'd been expecting to lose my job at any time. It wasn't nice seeing my closest friends on the playing staff having such a hard time as well. Steve Clarke took over for the match at home to Man Utd, which we lost 5-1. We badly needed a great manager and coach. I thought Steve could have been that man. I'd always got on well with him despite the internal feuds. He wasn't Freddy's target, though, and they didn't come any bigger in the eyes of the Geordies than the gentleman who was introduced to the press as Ruud's replacement: Bobby Robson.

Chapter 12

Bobby Robson Arrives

BOBBY ROBSON: what a man. With him there was no question whether he 'got' the North East because he *was* the North East. The atmosphere immediately changed just by his being there. He didn't have to do anything, just be Bobby. His calming presence released a lot of pent-up stress among the players and staff. This was a high-status manager who had done most things in the game, very well. He had no need to throw his weight around, and by just being his natural, charming self he endeared himself to anyone he spoke to. He made sure that he spent time with all the staff. He wanted to know where we were from, what school we went to, names of spouses and children, etc.

As I got to know Bobby, we would often talk about the Langley Park and Stanley areas (which are beside each other, separated by farmers' fields). He knew about minor details; he was interested in my playing days, so I mentioned that I'd played a few games for South Moor Juniors before going to Arsenal. He knew local football so well that he immediately came back and said what a great little club it had been over the years. He didn't mention his own achievements other than to talk about things that might have been more relevant to me, such as his playing and managing days at our mutual club, Fulham. It was never long until the conversation came back to home and the love he had for the region and the people. Such a humble man.

He told me that, although Newcastle was always his team, he would go to watch Sunderland play on free weekends when Newcastle were playing away. This was another time period while I was at the club when Geordie pride manifested itself. Bobby was the first to declare his love for the region he grew up in. He was a Geordie despite being born in Sacriston, just north of Durham, exemplifying that those who called themselves Geordie did so partly because of where they were born, but also because of their connection through growing up in this mining area, the accent and often working-class upbringing.

* * *

At times when people like Bobby talk about their connection to this region, it makes you think, *What creates this sense of pride in our community?* Part of it's a perception of being slightly isolated from the rest of England and the UK, while at the same time having an amazing history. How can that be? We're not isolated, are we? Well, first of all, to the east there's a 100 miles of coastline between Berwick and Hartlepool. What a maritime and riparian heritage we have as a result: St Aidan coming to Lindisfarne and restoring Christianity to England, then the Vikings raiding the same Holy Island; centuries later, mariners traded in silks, gin and amber with the Baltic merchants of the Hanseatic League. Then there's our modern history of the mines, with keelmen bringing the coal, the 'black diamonds' down the mighty rivers of Tyne and Wear to the waiting colliers to take coal *from* Newcastle, of course; tax on the coal, most of it coming from Newcastle, one shilling per chaldron (ton), helped rebuild St Paul's Cathedral after the Great Fire of London. At one point, the northern coalfield was the greatest producer of coal by volume in the world. The rivers developed into great industrial hubs. We took great pride in our shipbuilding. Mining, shipbuilding and steel put us at the heart of the Industrial Revolution. Most of that's now in the past, but the community remains.

Away from the coast and rivers to the north of Newcastle, once you get past Ashington, there's not a lot of people. Beautiful countryside and rich agriculture, but not many people. The same goes for the other side of the border until you get to Edinburgh. We have the border reivers to thank for that. For hundreds of years, given licence by kings, families and clans raided across the border, stealing whatever they could. If you stood in their way you would be killed. As a result, it was not a particularly nice place to live. Many people left. Those that remained had to be hardy types. The border lands to this day are still relatively empty.

To the west there are the Pennine Hills and to the south the Yorkshire Dales, Cleveland Hills and North York Moors. These areas were historically inhospitable places to live, so few people live there either. The empty areas cannot be talked about without mentioning Hadrian's Wall, stretching from Wallsend to the Solway, through some of the remotest terrain in Britain. Going there today is still an amazing experience, just to see the otherworldly Great Whin Sill landscape that's home to the wall. It's not difficult to imagine being a Roman soldier standing in the same place 2,000 years ago. Probably loving the summers and hating the winters. The area of the wall to the west is pretty wild, but the same wall that crosses through wildness goes through Newcastle too. There's even a Roman temple in the middle of a Benwell housing estate!

Most of us who live in the North East today are crammed into the great conurbation, from Ashington to Middlesbrough, but never too far inland from the coast. We're definitely a part of England, but just a bit isolated from the rest of it! Actor Kevin Bacon is linked to the concept of 'Six Degrees of Separation'. This 'law' says that any two people in the Hollywood film industry can be linked to one another via acquaintance with Kevin through film roles in six steps. Anywhere in the North East we have more of a subconscious perception of 'Three Degrees of Separation' from *anybody*. How many times in conversation do we attempt to find that connection with each other?

* * *

Back to football, people might be surprised at how organised Bobby was. He sat Paul and me down and said he would leave all decisions about player fitness to us. All he asked was that the injured players worked hard, doing two sessions, morning and afternoon. He was the first manager who implemented a daily morning medical meeting with the doc, physios and himself. This organisation was apparent in everything he did. Although he had coaches, Bobby was the *head* coach. Despite being 66, he would participate in training and playing while doing the coaching. After training he insisted that the players remained and had their lunch at the training ground. There was no 'popping to McDonald's on the way home from training' for Bobby. In the canteen, Bobby had the tables arranged in order. He would inspect and taste the food and chat with Liz the chef and then only allow one table up at a time to get their food. When the lads had finished eating, he would stand up and give a little talk, perhaps about how well they'd trained, or something about an upcoming match. He would then allow the lads to leave. He clearly revelled in the role, but the message was: 'Winning football matches is a serious matter.'

His first match in charge was away to Chelsea. It was 17 years since he'd last managed an England club team: Ipswich. We lost 1-0, but both sets of fans gave him a great reception, which was lovely to see. He was genuinely touched by the affection the supporters had for him. That was a thing about him, he was always pleasantly surprised if someone gave him a compliment. He told us that it was almost 50 years earlier that he started his football career, just down the road at Craven Cottage. Furthermore, it was also 50 years since his home was the North East. Despite that, Newcastle United was always his club and this place was always his spiritual home.

The result at Stamford Bridge meant we had one point out of a possible 21. We didn't care. To us it was inevitable that this squad of players would start performing and pick up the points. His first home match in charge was against Sheffield Wednesday. It was another of those days for the history books. It was a party atmosphere hours before kick-off and the occasion was matched by the result: 8-0. We blew Wednesday away that day. Alan scored five. I wonder if Ruud watched the game on satellite TV somewhere. From then on we did well, especially at home. We managed to get through to the third round of the UEFA Cup, beating CSKA Sofia and FC Zürich on the way. At the end of November we went down by a single goal away to Roma, when Laurent Charvet mistimed his tackle in the box, giving them a penalty. In the return leg we were convinced our momentum would see us through, but we only managed a 0-0 draw at St James' and it was over. What a frustrating 90 minutes that was.

We also had another Wembley trip, but this was a semi-final. It was against Chelsea. We went in with some good form behind us. We knew we had some great players in the team capable of beating them. We went in 1-0 down at half-time. After the restart

Alan did some great work down the right wing and hit an inch-perfect cross for Rob to power in a header. The Toon supporters went crazy. After that it looked as if we were going to press on and get the winner. Against the run of play, Poyet managed to loop a header over Shay and into the net. That was that: another Wembley defeat. This one was just as hard to take as the finals. In the league we finished in 11th place. The last match was a bit of a party atmosphere at St James' when we beat Arsenal 4-2 and Alan scored the 300th goal of his career, smashing a free kick through the Arsenal wall. The good times were back at the Toon and everyone was looking forward to next season.

We started 2000/01 well. At home the stadium had been refurbished and extended again, so there were now 52,000 fans to look forward to every match. We were told Bobby had very little money to spend on players because of the amount spent on the ground, which caused some disquiet among the supporters. It didn't help when Alan picked up another injury. This time it was his knee. He had a niggle that was made worse in an England friendly against Malta. He managed to get through the Euro 2000 competitions, but then missed a lot of matches. Despite that, we won three of the first four, followed by a series of mixed results.

We had to deal with several injuries at the time, including defenders Nikos Dabizas, Warren Barton and Marcelino (Martha as some of the lads called him). Martha had been in and out of the team with injury since Ruud bought him. The press didn't seem to mind when we had plenty of defenders such as Steve Howey and Laurent Charvet. But they'd been sold and we were short of centre-backs. The press really went for Martha, citing a 'finger injury' that kept him out for two months. They wrote their pieces as if it was as innocuous as a broken fingernail but he'd actually ruptured a flexor tendon when he snagged his finger on someone's shirt while making a challenge. He required surgery followed by a splint. The hand surgeon was quite clear: if he played too soon, he would re-rupture the tendon. I think the criticism he came in for during that period did have an adverse psychological effect on him. Shortly after that he played his final match for the first team and went into the reserves. He was eventually sold to a Spanish club.

We were still training down at the Riverside in Chester-le-Street. Those of us who lived south of the river would usually catch the train for away matches in London at Durham station. I had many interesting conversations with Bobby standing on that platform waiting for the Edinburgh to King's Cross express. He would be at his philosophical best. Once a train came screaming through the station. Bobby watched it fly by: 'How does a train stay on the track, Derek?'

'What?'

'The track. How does a train stay on the track when it's travelling so fast like that, on a bend?'

I thought for a while. 'I think it's something to do with the shape of the wheels.'

'Wheels? Tiny things like that? No, why does it stay on the track on a bend?'

I thought some more. 'Isn't it to do with physics?'

'Physics?'

'Aye, physics. Isn't it gravity, and the faster the train goes the more it sticks to the line?'

'No, but how does gravity stop it falling off?'

'What about centrifugal force? The faster the train goes, the harder the force on the rail keeping it on. Plus, the train tilts a bit.'

'Aye, it did tilt. But how does centrifugal force stop a train falling off the tracks on a bend at high speed?'

'No idea, Bobby.'

'Weird, isn't it?'

'Aye.'

Another time, he'd just made a phone call to New Zealand. 'Derek, aren't phones amazing? I've just made a phone call to New Zealand. How is that even possible?'

I thought for a while. 'Satellites, Bobby.'

'What?'

'Satellites. That's how you can make a call to New Zealand.'

'Aye, satellites.' He stood and contemplated for a while. 'Derek, what makes satellites stay in the sky? I mean, why don't they just fly off into space or just crash down to Earth?'

'Isn't it to do with how fast they go?'

'What's that got to do with it?'

'Well, if they go too fast, they'll fly off, and if they go too slow, they'll crash. Gravity and all that.'

'Aye, gravity is what makes them crash, but why do they just keep going round and round?'

'No idea, Bobby. It's physics.'

'I know, weird isn't it?'

'Aye.'

* * *

Something else Bobby commented on frequently was his pride in our military and in particular the North East regiments. He was prevented from doing National Service because of partial deafness, something he regretted. The achievements of the fighting men from the North East seems to have been forgotten. Doing some research, I was taken aback. In both world wars and earlier, the North East provided more conscripts to the army, per head, than anywhere else in England. The people also bought more war bonds for the cause than anywhere else. The division with the most fighting experience in the Second World War was the 50th Northumbrian, which comprised the Northumberland and Durham Regiments as well as soldiers from north and east Yorkshire. As D-Day approached, Montgomery insisted that the elite 50th Division was at the front. They were some of the last off the beaches of Dunkirk; in fact, men of the Durham Light Infantry (DLI) were the only soldiers of the expeditionary force to make the German army, an SS division in this case, withdraw temporarily in panic. Many in the DLI were miners. They had a reputation for being extremely fit. They fought ruthlessly in silence because they'd learned to conserve their voice while at the coalface. Montgomery said this of the DLI:

> It is a magnificent regiment. Steady as a rock in battle and absolutely reliable on all occasions. The fighting men of Durham are splendid soldiers; they excel in the hard-fought battle and they always stick it out to the end; they have gained their objectives and held their positions even when all their officers have been killed and conditions were almost unendurable.

It isn't just the 20th Century, this proud history goes way back. I think nearly all of us younger than Bobby's generation have forgotten this part of our history, so I'm grateful that he and his generation do remind us about this from time to time.

* * *

February through to mid-April 2001 weren't good for the team and we continued to deal with a lot of injuries, including Kieron, who was having a problem with recurring shin splints, but Bobby steadied the ship and once again we finished 11th. A lot of supporters considered that to be a failure. I think it was down to the expectations we all had at the start of the season. It wasn't a coincidence that Alan missed a lot of matches and only scored seven goals in all competitions.

In the close season, Kieron had surgery for the stress fracture of his leg and was able to rehab over the window. Bobby brought in Craig Bellamy and Laurent Robert. Bobby had tried to get Bellas the season before, when he was at Norwich. That fell through and the Welshman had gone to Coventry. He finally got his man, with a £6m price tag. He proved to be worth every penny. Mick Wadsworth left to go to Southampton and Bobby promoted John Carver to be the first-team coach. JC was great for Bobby and the team, injecting lots of quality positive coaching mixed with passion. He had good analytical skills and was able to assess the opposition well, then suggest in a clear and concise manner how their strong and weak points could be dealt with. I think Bobby liked that. It meant he could step back a little from coaching and get on with being manager and motivating the lads, and leave the technical side to JC, knowing it was being attended to in a professional manner. He also finally got his wish to move the training from the Riverside. He used to say that the infrastructure was inadequate: the first-team pitches were excellent, but the reserves' pitch wasn't as good and there were no other facilities. The club had finally acquired Darsley Park in Benton, but while that area was being prepared we moved to Blue Flames, which was beside it. The facilities there were excellent, and Bobby loved it there.

We started 2001/02 with two draws. The first was away to Chelsea with their big-buy stars, then it was 1-1 at home to the Mackems. For the next match, Alan returned from injury and we had a great 4-1 win away at Boro. Bellas ran their defence ragged, creating the space for Alan. Then came one of those matches many Toon supporters remember: the rollercoaster at home to Man Utd on 15 September. It was Bobby's 100th match in charge. Laurent Robert was great that day. He smashed the first goal in from a free kick. Then they got one back through Ruud van Nistelrooy. They had all the stars: Beckham, Giggs, Cole and Keane in midfield, with some impressive periods controlling the play. Never mind that, what a team we had: Nobby Solano, Alan, Rob, Bellas. Such great skill, with speed up front. Bellas was constantly threatening, with Rob Lee the rock as always. In the second half we went 3-1 up through Rob and Nikos Dabizas. These were Bobby's entertainers. It should be Bobby's Dazzlers really. Such skill, and what a difference pace makes to a team.

They weren't finished, being a Ferguson team; they fought their way back to 3-3, first through a Giggs goal on the hour then, straight after, from Verón. Perhaps it was going the way of so many other matches we had against Man Utd? But no, not in Bobby's 100th match. Wes Brown helped Alan's header in to his own goal in the last ten minutes. Come the final minute, frustrating as it might be, Alan was running down the clock by the Strawberry corner of the Gallowgate End and Roy Keane lost the plot. All Alan had to do was stand his ground for Keane to see red … then see red. After the match ended, we made sure Alan wasn't going to do anything silly in the tunnel. Keane was waiting for him after the final whistle, surrounded by Man Utd staff, of course. Even if he really wanted to, there was no way we would have let him get to Alan, although Al can handle himself anyway.

But what a win. The city was bouncing that Saturday night in September. It really was some team. Alan was a goalscoring machine. The two youngsters, Bellas and Kieron, were exceptional in speed and skill. Gary Speed was a brilliant midfield rock for them: great discipline, organised, intelligent. And then there was Nobby, with his South American genius, so graceful on the ball and capable of beating defenders if called to do so, or releasing inch-perfect passes with impeccable timing. He was also an accomplished goalscorer. Nobby always had a smile on his face. He called me 'El Gordo', which he assured me means 'the beautiful one'. I never checked to see if he was telling the truth.

Not long after that, we beat Villa at home when Alan side-footed a volley past Schmeichel, one of his best goals. On that high, we went on a winter break to Malaga. We were staying near Marbella. We were told last-minute that there was a dinner in honour of Sir John. Some of the lads, including Bellas and Kieron, didn't get the message. They went out in Puerto Banús for food. As usually happens in these situations, they had a skinful and came back to the hotel too late for the organised meal. It became more of an issue than it should have been and they ended up being sent home early, much to the delight of the press. What escaped the tabloids was the massive session we had with some of the senior players after the dinner.

Once we'd returned to England, we picked up ten points from five matches then beat Arsenal at Highbury to go top. The Gunners weren't happy. There was talk of our revenge for the 1996 match when Dixon kicked lumps out of David Ginola, and when David finally retaliated he was sent off in one of the worst refereeing displays I've ever seen. Well, since they brought it up, yes it was revenge. Then came an away match at Leeds to cap that result. It was just before Christmas; the lads fought back from 3-1 down to win 4-3 against David O'Leary's star-studded team, with the likes of Rio Ferdinand, Harry Kewell, David Batty, Mark Viduka, Lee Bowyer and Robbie Fowler. They were looking to replace us at the top. We fought back from two goals down. Kieron was finally fully fit. He slotted a pass through for Nobby's last-minute winner. The travelling Toon army went crazy. That was such a great time. We lost a couple of times after that, but we were never far away from winning matches. Bobby brought in Sylvain Distin and Jermaine Jenas over the January window. Things were looking promising again.

To bring us down to earth we sold Rob Lee and Warren Barton to Derby early in 2002. I'd spent a lot of time with those two wonderful guys, both socially and professionally, and it was one of those moments when you knew things will never quite be the same. What a time to get rid of such great players, riding high in the Premier League. We were *always* balancing the books. However, Olivier Bernard had returned from loan to join Jermaine and Sylvain as quality replacements for my old friends. Speedo continued to be a rock in the centre of midfield, and now he had the starlets, Kieron and JJ, beside him, with killer forwards ahead of them.

Kevin Keegan brought Man City to St James' in January for the fifth round of the FA Cup. What a reception Kevin received. I saw him looking around the place in awe, soaking in the applause. I'm sure for a while he forgot he was the visiting manager. City were playing in the tier below but played well that night; they pushed us all the way, just as you would expect a Keegan team to do. Nobby got our winner on the hour. But what a struggle it was, even against a team down to ten men for an hour.

The lads beat the Mackems away at the end of February, and Nikos whipped his shirt off when he scored the winner, while Shay was majestic in goal; but a real disaster from that match was Bellas picked up a patellar tendon injury. It started as an acute injury (partial tendon tear) on one side, but gradually developed over weeks into a chronic bilateral issue. He was so important to the team. Players with skill and speed are priceless because they open up the opposition for the rest of the team, either directly by getting into spaces ahead of the defenders, or by making them drop off, playing more of a negative game. Losing him at that point meant a lot. He joined Kieron on the treatment table. He was struggling with a stress fracture in his foot. We then lost two big matches in March, first home to Arsenal then away to Liverpool. Dennis Bergkamp scored his wonder goal against us for the Gunners, one of the best I've ever seen. He flicked it one way, around Nikos, ran the other way then met up with the ball he'd passed to himself and slid it past Shay. After the Liverpool match we had some good wins but had too many draws and just seemed to run out of matches, finishing in fourth place, six points behind Man Utd. Still, not bad, and it meant we had the same qualifying reward as them: a Champions League place for the following season. Craig Bellamy deservedly won the PFA Young Player of the Year Award for 2002. There was a lot of positive energy. Everyone knew Bobby was a great boss and he had a wonderful team. We were very optimistic for the following season.

Chapter 13

Bobby Robson 2

THE 2002/03 season started with us qualifying for the group stages of the Champions League, drawing Juventus, Dynamo Kyiv and Feyenoord in the first stage. In the league opener we had a good home win against West Ham, but we then went on a poor run, picking up only one point from four matches. We did follow that with three wins, though, starting with a 2-0 home victory against Sunderland.

We lost our first three Champions League matches in September and October so things were looking bleak for that competition. The press kept telling us no team had ever qualified from that position. We were still misfiring in the league when we went into the home match against Juventus. Nikos and Bellas were suspended and Bobby dropped Shay in favour of Harps. The lads battled hard for a deserved 1-0 victory, although we had a very tense last ten minutes when they seemed to be constantly pressing for the equaliser.

The next match, at the end of October, against Dynamo Kyiv at St James', was another must-win game. We went 1-0 down, but we knew the lads were always in this one. They kept plugging away. First, Speedo notched a header and then Alan scored the winner from the penalty spot.

What a match the away tie in Rotterdam against Feyenoord was, one of our great European nights. We needed to win, and Juve had to get a result against Dynamo for us to progress. Bellas had been to the US for surgery during the window and it was great to have him finally back in the team, linking with Speedo, Kieron, JJ and Al. The team were on fire. We were 2-0 up early in the second half, but they drew level with 20 minutes to go. Tommo was keeping us up to date with the score in Kyiv. Just when we were on the ropes and resigning ourselves to a UEFA Cup place, Bellas pounced on a parried shot from Kieron and put us through to the next group stage. What a celebration! The whole bench was up and on the pitch. That is, except King Bobby. He sat on the bench, beaming in delight. 'Calm down, lads, calm down,' he said, grinning like the Cheshire cat.

In November, a week after the Feyenoord match, Bobby was knighted: Sir Bobby. Well deserved.

He remained down to earth, though. After home matches he would come into the physios' room and sit and chat with whoever was there. My dad was usually there, waiting for me to finish off and to get a lift home. Bobby would often sit and discuss the match with him, using plastic cups or cans of lager to explain players' positions for set pieces, etc. On occasion, Bobby would also get his hair cut in there while chatting away to us. A woman always came down from one of the kitchens with a tray of lamb chops cooked in mint sauce for him. He would eat a couple and carefully wrap the remaining ones in aluminium foil to take home for later. Ah, happy days.

Bobby was such a funny guy. I remember once I was talking to Steve Taylor when he was recovering from an injury. Things weren't progressing as quickly as we wanted, so I told him we would check his electrolytes. I later walked past Sir Bobby, who was talking to one of the coaches, saying, 'Derek is popping round to Steven's later to check on his electric lights.'

We were soon playing the second phase of the Champions League. We took a beating at home from Inter after playing most of the match down to ten men when Craig Bellamy was sent off following some 'professional play' by the defender Marco Materazzi. Our Welshman reacted to Materazzi's challenge (and surreptitious pinching of his skin, something totally alien to the British game) and the Italian international made it look as bad as he possibly could. It ended 4-1, an awful night all round.

In the league, we'd started the season slowly, but the home win over the Mackems started a good run of form. At the beginning of December, four days after the loss to Inter, Alan scored a superb goal in the 2-1 win at home to Everton. They'd been rampant in the league before that. We were 1-0 down with six minutes left when Alan hit an unstoppable volley from 22 yards. Shola headed up a ball, Alan hit it on the volley, top right corner. Then, with two minutes left, Bellas popped up with his deflected decider, winning back the hearts of the Geordies after his sending-off.

The next match was a 3-1 defeat at the Camp Nou, so that was the first two matches we'd lost in the second phase of the Champions League. At least in the league we started picking up a lot of points and playing with quality. Bobby signed Jonathan Woodgate from Leeds in January. The lad could be a bit of a character off the pitch, but he was a fantastic centre-half. We took six points off Leverkusen in the Champions League, then had the away trip to Milan. That was another great match, in the San Siro. There were 12,000 Geordies massed inside, with their St George's crosses and Union Jacks draped across the barriers. What an atmosphere they created.

Let's see how we do with 11 of Bobby's Dazzlers on the pitch compared with the ten-man team we had at St James, I thought. We led twice. The Italians had all the theatrics, like going to ground every time they were in the box. Once they equalised, they held on, but the lads did themselves proud fighting to get a winner. We ran out of time and that draw meant we had to win our final match at home to Barça and hope the Inter result went our way. The lads started great in that match too, blistering pace and incessant pressure. We failed to take a couple of chances. Then we heard that Inter were winning in Germany; that deflated us, and the Spaniards regained their composure. They took the lead on the hour, then we were chasing the game. They made in 2-0 towards the end. What a disappointment. It wasn't to be a repeat of the glory night Tino had against the Catalans six years earlier.

Although we hammered Blackburn 5-1 at home only three days later, that result didn't reflect the disappointment that pervaded the whole club. The Champions League exit had taken the wind out of our sails in the league. We lost away to Everton then the next home match was at home to Man Utd on 12 April. JJ scored first, but in the last 12 minutes of the first half they tore us apart, putting four past us. They started the second half as they ended the first, and with more than half an hour left to go they'd scored six. Some of the fans walked out, before Shola pulled one back near the end. We knew then that our chance of winning the league that season had gone. We lost away to Fulham and drew at home to Villa but then had a great away win against Sunderland when Nobby's penalty separated the teams. We finished the season in third with an away draw with West Brom, but a long way behind Man Utd and Arsenal. But that meant another qualifying round place in the Champions League. The fans were happy, as we were making progress: fourth to third in successive seasons. JJ won the PFA Young Player of the Year Award.

The 2003/04 season got off to a bad start. Lee Bowyer was the only player we brought in during the summer break. We went out of the Champions League qualifying rounds at the first hurdle. We beat Partizan Belgrade in the away tie 1-0, but lost at home by the same scoreline, forcing it to penalties. It was 2-2 after the first round of ten penalties, both teams failing to score three penalties each. Even Alan missed one for us. It then went to sudden death. JJ scored, they scored. Aaron Hughes missed but they scored, knocking us out. That was tough to take. As Bobby said to the press, everyone was distraught. That word summed it up. He was very gracious in defeat as he always was, praising the Serbians on their hard-fought victory.

Some events have a symbolic meaning and this felt like one of those times: almost but not quite doing it the season before, rumours of a lack of money for players then an early departure from a massive competition this time round. Had our momentum under Bobby peaked? We lost at home to Birmingham after the Champions League exit, following that with two draws, then a 3-2 loss at Highbury on 26 September. It was a Friday night match and some of the lads stayed down in London for a night out. An incident occurred in the Grosvenor House Hotel. Some of the team were accused of rape. The press had yet another field day. Kieron had all sorts of allegations made against him and he wasn't even involved! It took many months for this to end in nothing, with no one charged, but it certainly put a strain on the lads involved, and Bobby as their manager came in for criticism.

On the pitch, we didn't get our first league win until the beginning of October. However, by the end of that month we'd won four times in the league and progressed to the second round of the UEFA Cup. We continued doing well as we ended the year. We went to Vålerenga in Norway for the third round, first leg of the UEFA Cup. Bobby left Alan out of the team. Alan wasn't happy about that. He had words with Sir Bobby. That was disquieting. The lads brought a draw back and we beat them at St James' at the beginning of March. After a win at home to Charlton a couple of weeks later, we were in fifth place.

In the last week of March we went to Mallorca for the fourth round, second leg tie of the UEFA Cup, having already won 4-1 at home. That was when Bellas and JC had their bust-up in Newcastle airport. I wasn't there, so Ferra was covering that match. It was to do with Bellas nicking John Carver's parking space at the training ground for a laugh. When JC finally confronted him about it at the airport, they started rucking on the floor. Bobby was trying to do a press interview, separated by a screen, but the ruction brought that to an abrupt halt. The fight on the way to Spain didn't affect the lads: they won 3-0. Alan scored two and Bellas one.

There was a change in mood about the club at this time. It was difficult to put your finger on why, but one factor might have been *Goal*. The directors had allowed this movie production to be filmed in and around the stadium and training ground. It was produced by Touchstone Pictures (Walt Disney Studios) with the blessing of FIFA. It had a substantial marketing contribution (fee) from Adidas. Bobby was told to ask the lads if they would allow the film's crew to train and play with them, interact with them and generally blend into their day-to-day life while training or playing. The players hated the idea. They didn't want outsiders getting into their inner sanctum of the training ground, changing room and playing field. It caused a rift with some of the players. The lads eventually got their way, and the production team were kept at arm's-length. I kept my head down, but I do remember treating the lead actor's Achilles tendon injury! It was a strange time and it coincided with rumours circulating that Sir Bobby had 'lost the dressing room'.

In April we squeezed past PSV in the quarter-finals of the UEFA Cup. We'd drawn 1-1 in the first leg but Alan and Speedo got the goals at St James' in the second leg 2-1 win. Laurent Robert was on fire again that match, and PSV struggled to cope with his deliveries. That meant the Toon's first last-four place in a senior European competition in 35 years. We were rewarded with a semi-final tie against Marseille. We took a few injuries into the first leg at home on 20 April. That was a tough encounter; we were unable to get the breakthrough, while Didier Drogba always threatened to score for them. Jonathan Woodgate had a great match, though, and it finished goalless. The return was at the beginning of May. A lot of the guys were injured, including Bellas, JJ and Woody. Before kick-off, the dreaded cast from *Goal* were filming beside the lads, to look as if they were the ones warming up before playing. The players still objected to that. They felt that the bosses hadn't listened to their requests. Sir Bobby had obviously been pressurised from upstairs to allow it. But that didn't stop the senior players voicing their opinions once more. Of course, there was no Freddy Shepherd or Hall Jr there to listen to that, so Sir Bobby got it in the neck.

Marseille's ground, the Vélodrome, was a good size, but they'd packed in the supporters. The attendance that day, nearly 59,000, broke the club's record. Hardly any Toon fans were given tickets. Perhaps their directors had seen the effect 12,000 Geordies had in Milan the year before. The French supporters certainly succeeded in making it an intimidating experience. We had to stop halfway through the first half when the police dealt with flares thrown on the pitch. It was another tight affair, but two Drogba goals sunk us. Once again, we were close but ultimately unsuccessful in the 2-0 defeat. There was a sense of inevitability about it.

We felt dejected and weary heading into the remaining league fixtures. In the penultimate home match Alan scored a screamer against Chelsea in the 2-1 win. Olivier passed it up to him on the left wing, some way off the angle of the 18-yard box. He was being marked by Desailly, but by just backing into him then twisting and stepping on to his left foot, it gave Alan plenty of space to launch the ball into the top right corner. The final match at home to Wolves ended as a disappointing 1-1 draw. The chance of us finishing fourth, above Liverpool and in a Champion's League spot, receded with the two dropped points.

We drew our final two away matches and finished fifth, four points behind Liverpool, not quite good enough for a Champion's League spot. However, we qualified for the UEFA Cup, but having had a taste of the Champions League, to many fans this was viewed as a negative. There was an awful feeling of anticlimax about the season. We'd gone from finishing 11th twice, to fourth, then third but now finished fifth. Some considered that failure. Once again, I began to worry for the incumbent manager: Sir Bobby. I believed he was the best chance we had for success and he had a great coach in JC. We would be able to sort out the injuries and get the senior players fit again. All he needed was the funding to bring in a couple of key players and we would have that winning opportunity.

Before the start of the new season, Freddy sold Jonathan Woodgate to Real Madrid. Sir Bobby wasn't involved in the sale; he deliberately went on record to say he didn't want him to go. Freddy said it was to enable the club to sign Wayne Rooney from Everton; we never landed Rooney. What he did for Man Utd is history. But we'd signed Patrick Kluivert earlier and were well off for forwards, so we were still confident that Sir Bobby would do well. However, the rumours continued to circulate that he'd lost the dressing room. I was frequently asked about this and denied any knowledge. But, privately, I had concerns. A couple of the young players were a bit of a handful and Bellas would sometimes backchat him, but he could start a fight in an empty room. Kieron and Sir Bobby got on well, but on occasion they would fall out too. There was also the hangover about the way the owner and chairman reacted to the European exit and the whole team's dissent about the *Goal* shenanigans. Still, I expected that the directors would stick with Bobby. He'd said one or two things to Ferra and me in passing that suggested he might be planning to step down at the end of the season, so we were hoping for one last shot at the title. It didn't help the situation when Freddy sold Speedo to Bolton. Gary was well respected in the dressing room. He always had Sir Bobby's back and the youngsters responded to his lead.

Then came the 2004/05 opener away to Boro. Kieron had been asked to play on the wing. He'd objected to that and discussed it with Sir Bobby; he was put on the bench. A lot of the lads were missing because of injuries and viral conjunctivitis. Despite that, we took the lead and we thought we'd won it, but they equalised at the death. Kieron apologised to Sir Bobby, but the news quickly spread that he'd 'refused to play'. Some blamed his absence for not winning. The manager was perceived by the press to have lost the ruthless streak a manager needs. The younger players were given the title 'The Brats' by the press. This wasn't justified at all, but there was perhaps a bit of a divide developing among the players. Nothing you could put your finger on. I think they were just a bit jaded, pissed off. There were two groups, the younger single lads and the older married lads. Not much of an issue. It happens.

Then we lost at home to Spurs in our first home match. It was an end-to-end entertaining affair, but they took the lead early in the second half and, although we had chances, we couldn't make the breakthrough. Kieron came on as a sub, and a section of the supporters booed him. That brought back some of the feelings from the preceding season's end. A sense of 'same old team, same old manager' appeared to be developing. Next came a home match against Norwich. Aaron scored early in the second half to make it 2-0, but they came straight back at us and scored, then equalised with 15 minutes to go. Another match where we gave away the lead. Ferra and I discovered Kieron sitting in the bath afterwards, long after all the others had left. He was pissed off with the situation, as we all were. Anything other than a victory resulted in negativity at that time. The board were super-sensitive to that.

Kieron had struggled in the Norwich match and the manager left him out of the squad for the away trip to Aston Villa. He put Alan on the subs bench, playing Patrick Kluivert instead. That match in Birmingham was another that we were winning but lost. Patrick played well, but by the time Alan came on and replaced him as sub it was too late to retrieve a point. Some supporters say Freddy signed a 'has-been' in Patrick, but he was only 28 when he arrived. He was expected to have two or three seasons at the top of his game. Anyway, it was always a risk to drop such a great striker as Alan, as Ruud had found out. Despite that decision, there was not quite the same sense of fatality when Sir Bobby did it, because he was so well respected. Having said that, some of the media were regularly reporting that his job was in jeopardy; reporters often knew things we didn't, so we did wonder among ourselves if something was happening.

The Villa match was played on 28 August and Freddy sacked Sir Bobby the next day. Ferra and I were at the training ground, treating some of the injured players. Ferra bumped into Sir Bobby sitting in the canteen alone, looking dishevelled and unhappy. He told Ferra that he'd been summoned to the ground and thought he would be gone. Ferra tried to reassure him. Sure enough, a couple of hours later he returned to clear out his office. We met him in the car park. He looked so sad, destroyed. Freddy later said it was like shooting Bambi. Sir Bobby looked as if one of his own family had been shot. We tried to comfort him, but what can you say? We told him he was loved by the Geordies and that he'd done a great job for the city and club. He briefly broke out in a smile, 'Do you think so?' he asked.

As I've said before, Bobby was always so humble and was genuinely surprised by a compliment. Of course, that's what we thought. A couple of the senior players were there, Steven Harper was one of them. There were some tears shed. We took some photos and helped him pack a couple of things, including a single golf club, in his car and that was that; he was gone. When Sir Bobby left, that ended arguably the fourth golden managerial period for Newcastle United: Stan Seymour Sr, Joe Harvey, Kevin Keegan, Sir Bobby Robson. It was undoubtedly the end of the second and final golden era that I was involved in at the club.

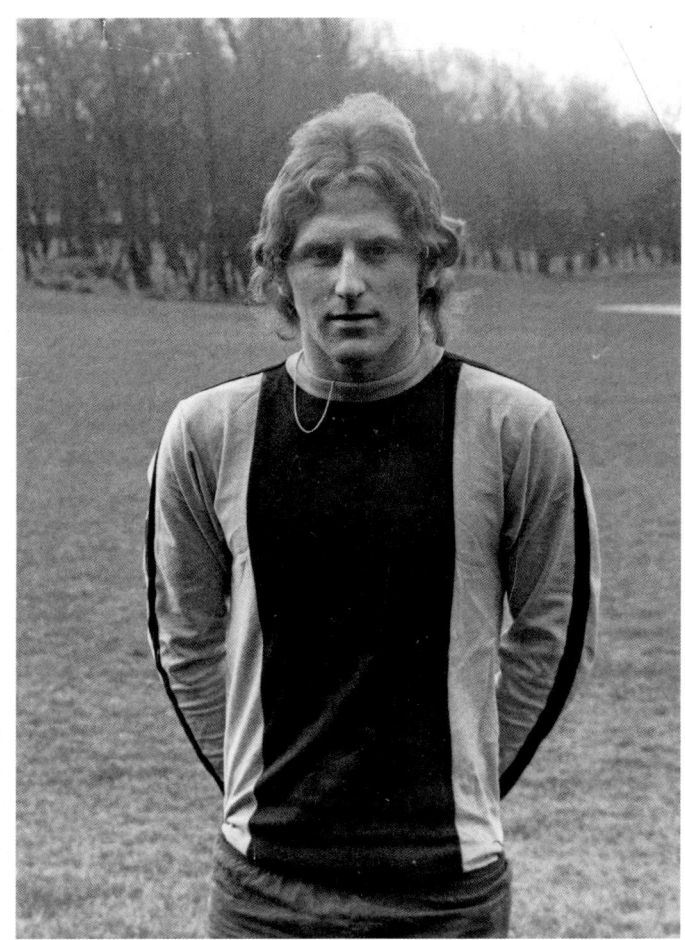

Tanfield school

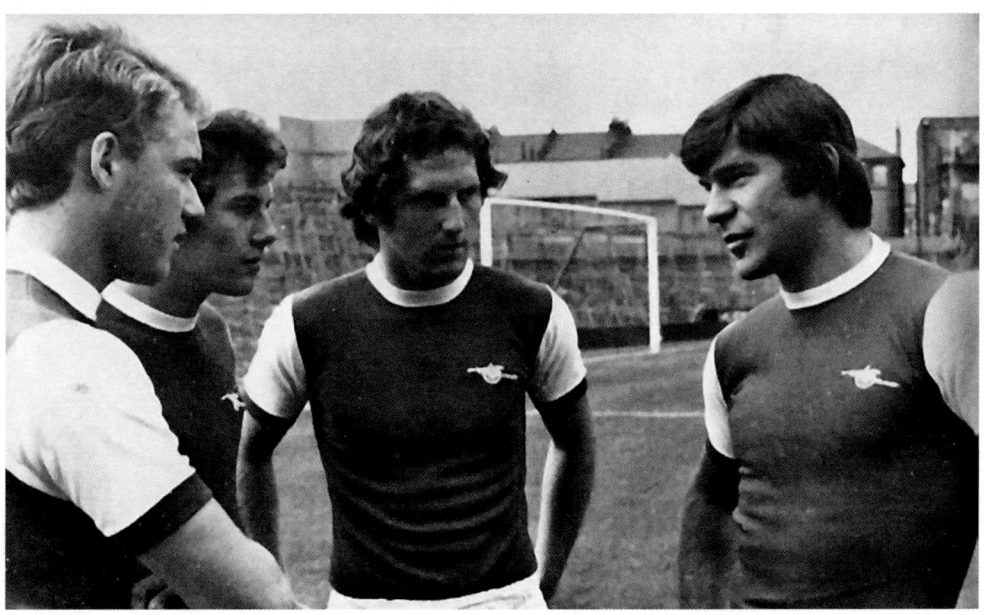

Apprentice at Arsenal. Pre-season, talking to Malcolm Macdonald

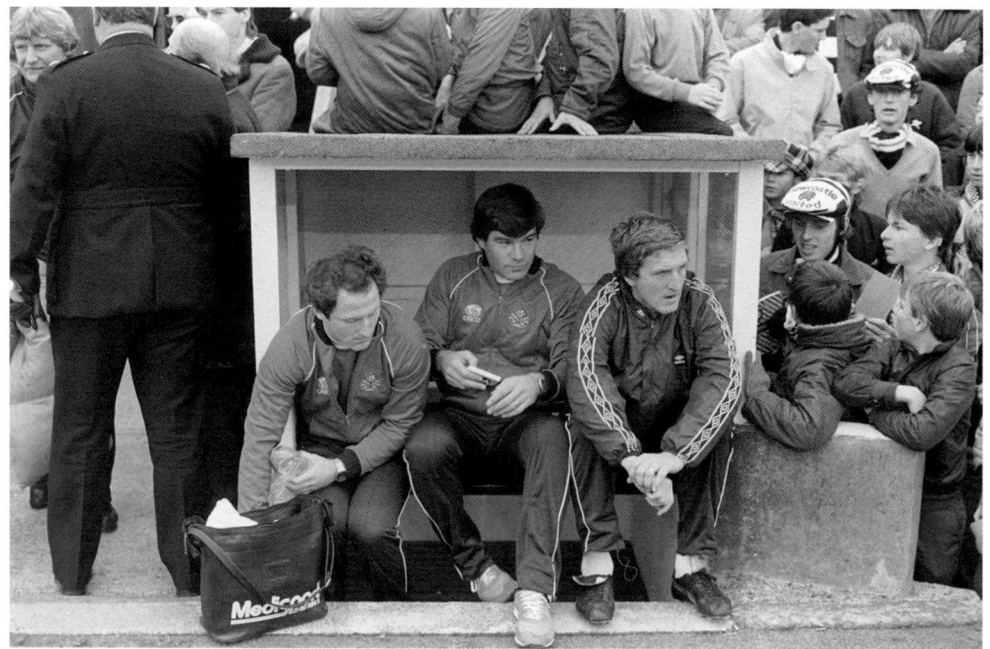

In the away dugout at St James' Park with Fulham: Malcolm Macdonald and Ray Harford

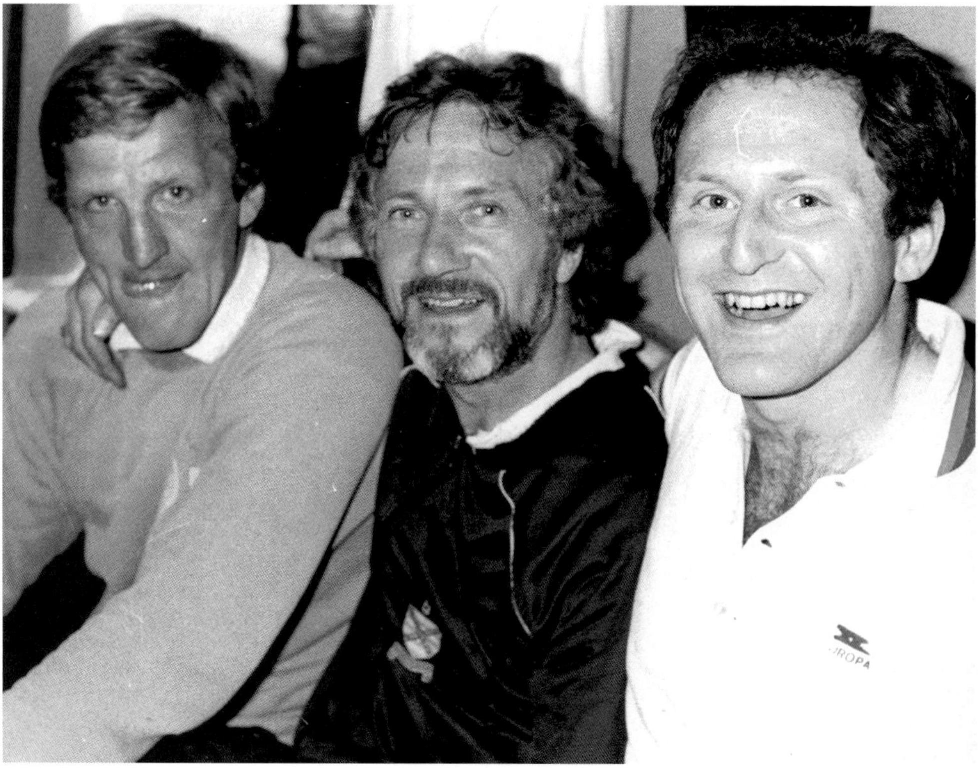

Just promoted from Division Three with Fulham. Ray Harford on the left and George Armstrong centre

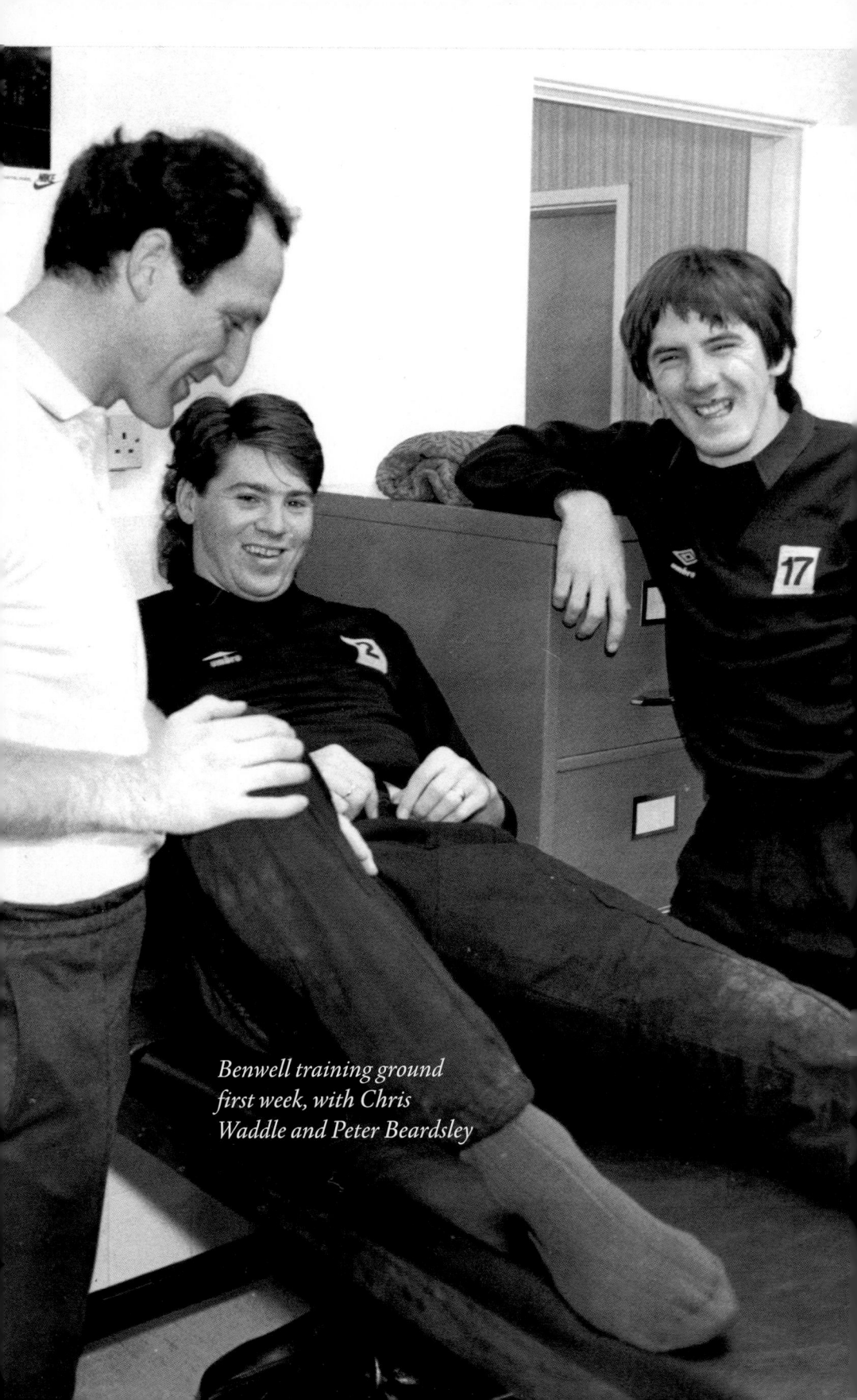

*Benwell training ground
first week, with Chris
Waddle and Peter Beardsley*

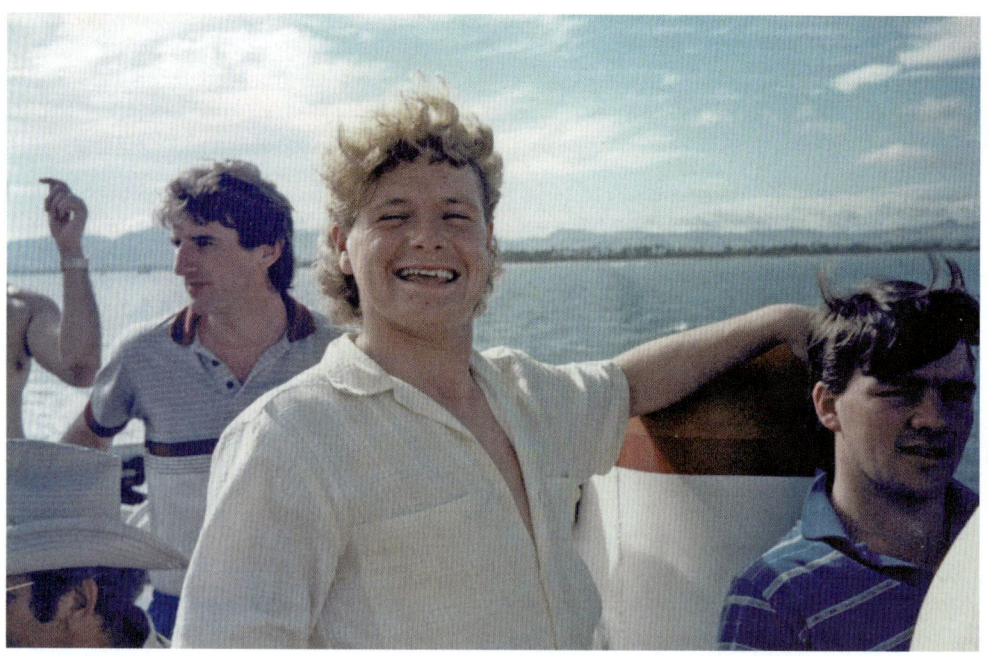

Tour of New Zealand. Gazza centre. John Anderson behind and Gary Kelly to Paul's left

Happy camper. Just played in the Isle of Man Tournament

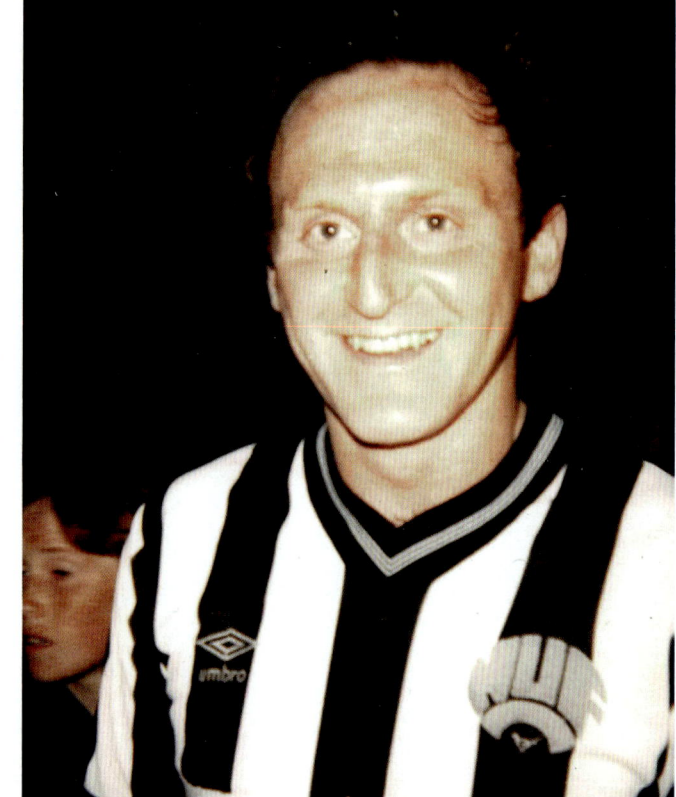

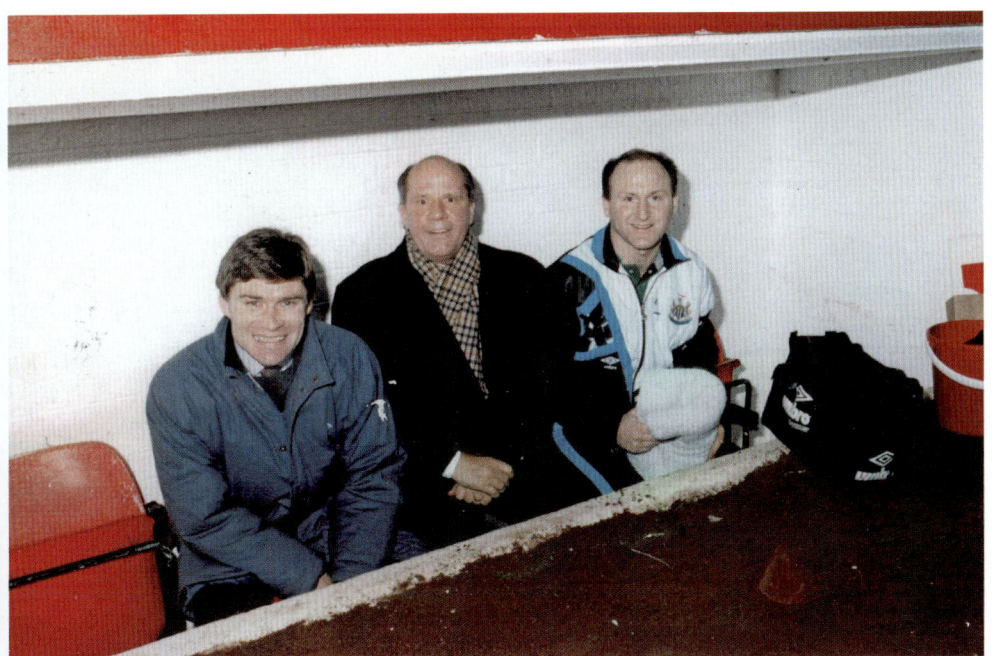

Derek Fazackerley left and Jim Smith centre

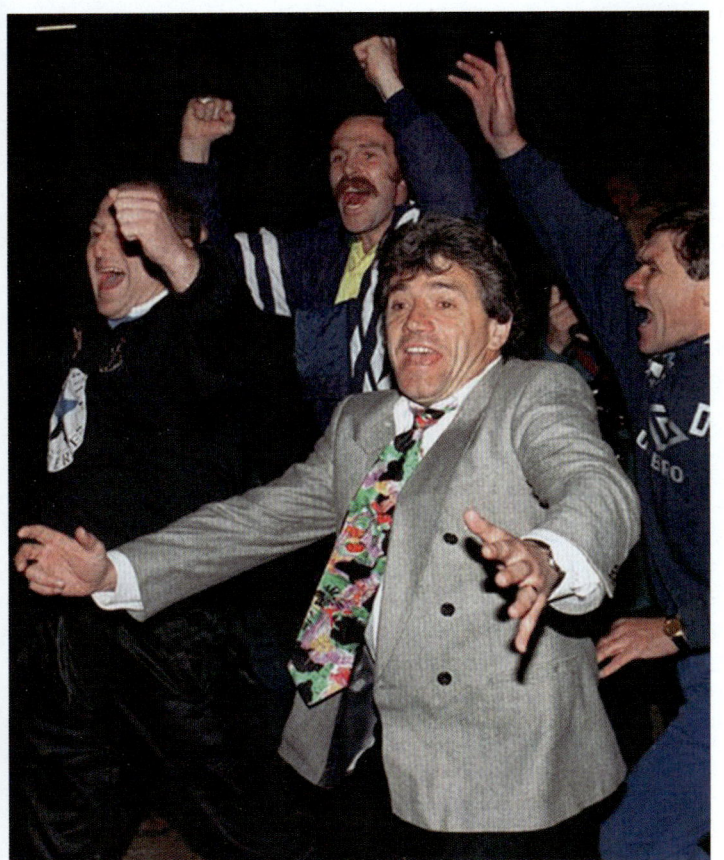

Clinching promotion at Grimsby. Kevin Keegan front, behind is Brian Kilcline and on Kevin's left is Derek Fazackerley

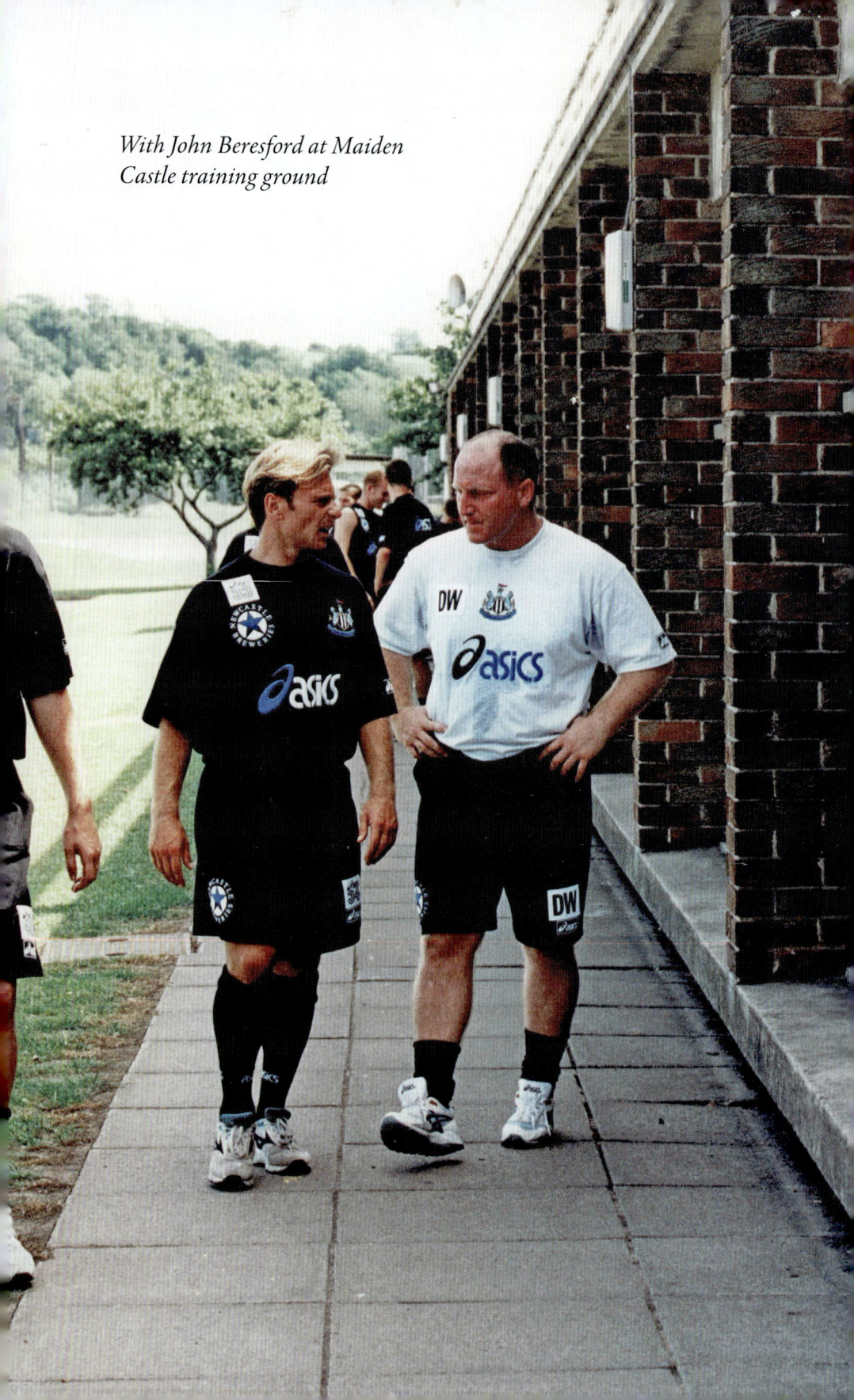

With John Beresford at Maiden Castle training ground

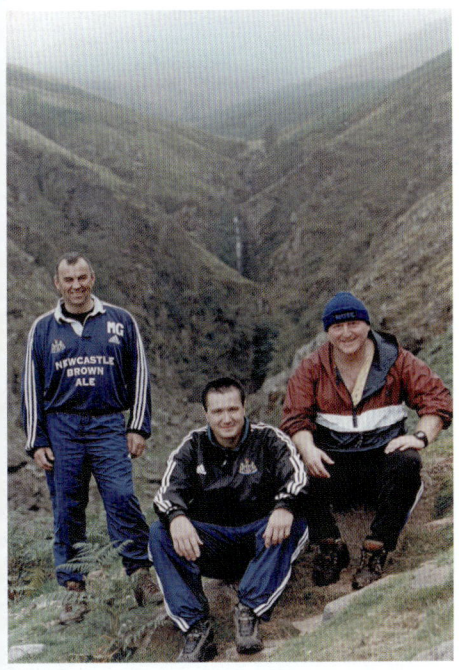

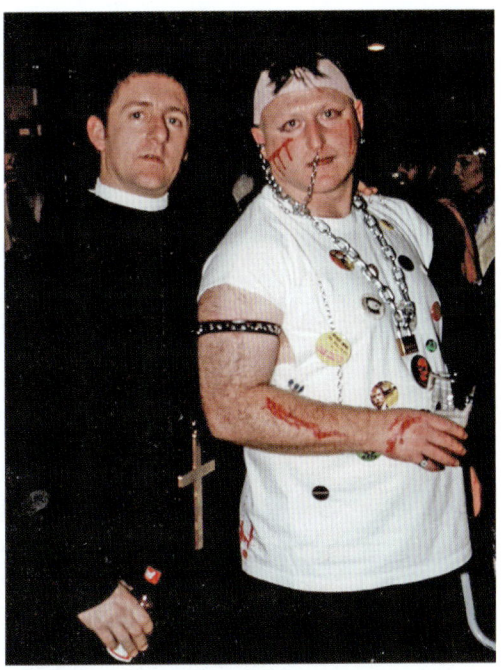

Rehab for Steve Howey in the Lake District Langdales. Masseur Mick Greener on Steve's right

Fancy dress party with Ray Thompson

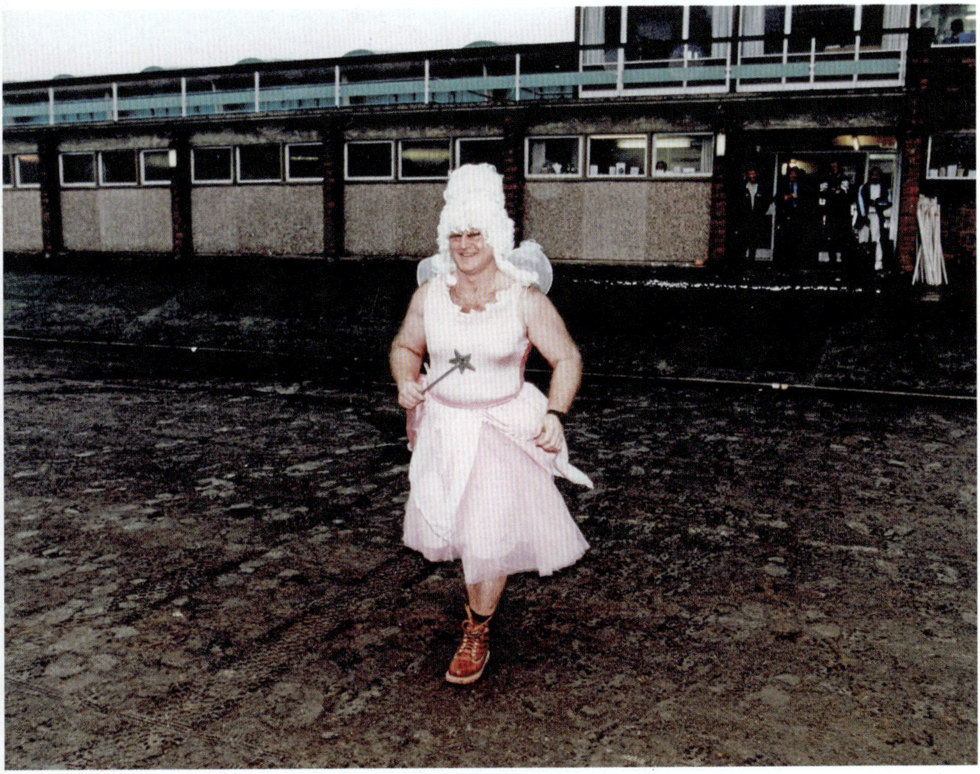

Pink fairy Christmas party. I'd just been bollocked by Kevin

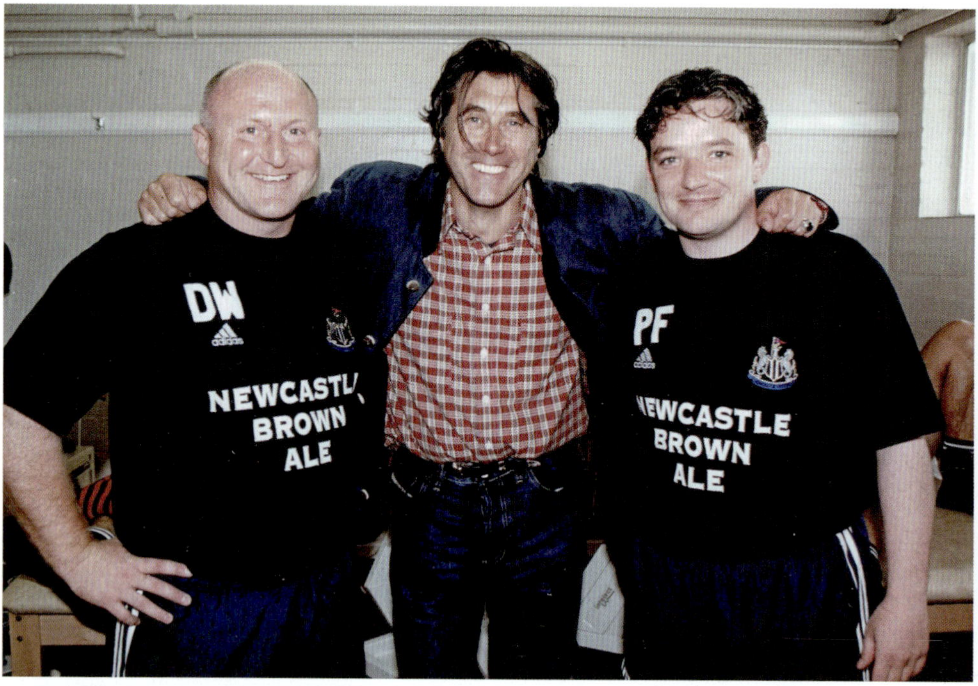

Bryan Ferry (centre) and Paul Ferris, Maiden Castle training ground

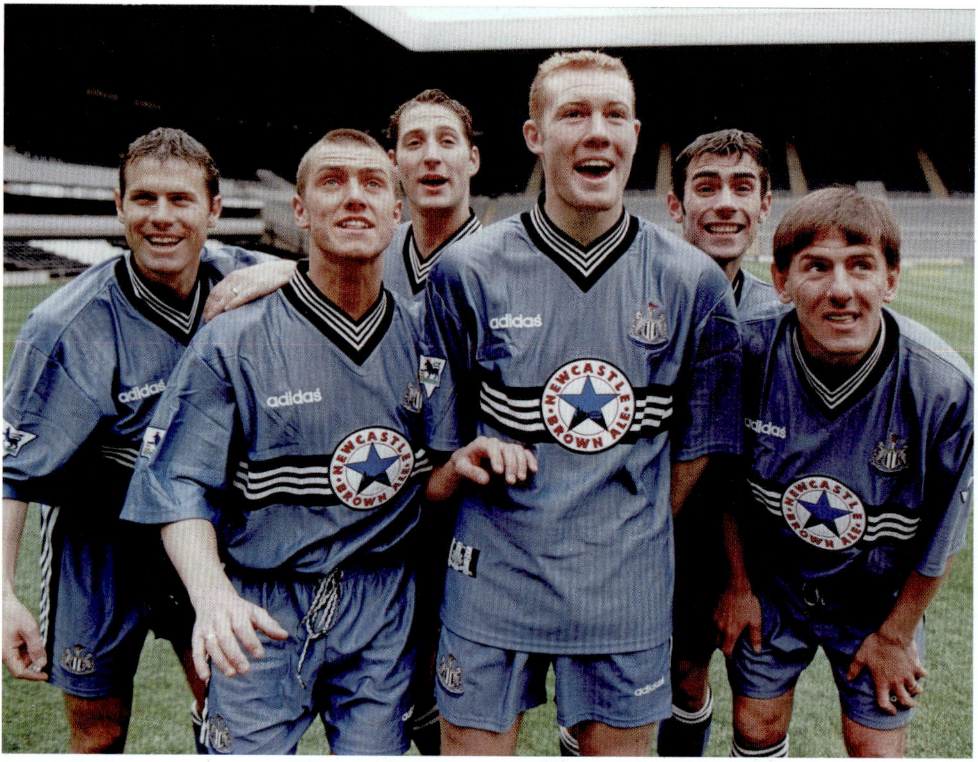

Some of the Entertainers team. Left to right: Rob Lee, Lee Clark, Robbie Elliott, Steve Watson, Keith Gillespie, Peter Beardsley

Chapter 14

Graeme Souness

FREDDY TOLD John Carver he was temporary manager until further notice. We got on with the job. JC was in charge for the home win against Blackburn on Saturday, 11 September. By then we knew Graeme Souness was taking over on the Monday. He watched from the stand as we beat the team he'd just left. It was a comfortable victory. We then went on to win three and get two away draws from the next five matches. That was followed by three defeats, including yet another home loss to Man Utd. Rooney scored one of the goals. Other than a good away win at Crystal Palace, we then had alternating draws and losses. On New Year's Day at home to Birmingham, the lads had a dominant victory, with Bellas in great form. He went off towards the end with an injury, though, joining Alan on the treatment bench.

Things were looking bright again. Away from the football, there had been a Christmas party at St James' for the staff. I was pleased to see Helen from the ticket office was there. She had a full-time job elsewhere but worked for the club part-time on matchdays. We always had a chat when I popped in to sort out the tickets for my dad. There was something about her, so I was pleased that she was at the party. I spent most of the evening talking to her and not long after that we started dating.

In the league we were doing okay at the start of 2005. Graeme had brought some staff with him. On the medical side he had Phil Boersma. Phil came across as a canny bloke. Graeme wanted him to be his rehab coach. He was a great player in his Liverpool days, but his knowledge base was lacking with regards to many aspects of physiotherapy and athletic performance. We weren't sure what a rehab coach was, but if rehab was mentioned it should come under medical, or be based on scientific knowledge. I asked Graeme if Phil was qualified for such a role. He told me that it didn't matter if he was qualified or not because that was his role for him. Fair enough, rehab coaches are definitely part of the game now.

By now, Ferra had had enough of being a professional football physio and was well down the path of self-improvement. In addition to funding his own physiotherapy education at university, he'd developed other skills. Over the preceding three years my colleague had studied diligently in the evenings. First, he did a master's in 'History of Ideas', then studied for a postgraduate law degree at the university by distance learning. That was a considerable effort required to learn a new profession. I had no idea how he found the time and energy to do it, because we had our hands full at the club.

I confined my education to sports medicine, attending a part-time course at Cardiff along with Kevin Bell, our new addition as a physiotherapist at the club, plus my brother, who attended as a doctor. The course was designed for physios and doctors and gave both sets of professionals a deeper insight into the developing speciality of sports medicine. The diploma consisted of course work, including two long weekends in Cardiff over the two years, followed by examinations. We met many interesting professionals on that course, including Steph Brennan. He was a very pleasant and knowledgeable Aussie physio working in professional rugby union in London.

Back at the club, the team continued picking up points and Graeme himself came across as a friendly but dominant character. Like his two ex-Liverpool team-mates who had been managers, he'd done everything in the game. That included a well-deserved reputation as a 'hard man' who never gave an inch to any opponent. He tackled the manager's job in the same way. Unfortunately, there are certain things in the manager's role that are out of your control; one of those was the injuries that piled up at this time. As a player all you can do is train harder and try to improve your attitude and technique. As a manager you have other individuals to deal with: players, medical staff, coaching staff and the directors. And that's not to mention the press and supporters. When it goes great, it must seem like the world is a lovely well-oiled machine, serendipitously providing you with all the victories you deserve with relatively little effort. When things go wrong, it must seem like the whole world is against you. *Why was that penalty given? Why does his injury keep breaking down? What's wrong with his attitude?* You get the picture. At that time, injuries were a problem for Graeme and for us.

Craig Bellamy had this knee issue, a genuine ongoing problem with his patellar tendon, but it was finally better. The manager had been arguing in the previous weeks with him about his best position to play. But one day, at the start of training, Bellas said he could feel his hamstring pulling. It became an issue for Graeme when one or two of the senior pros told him that Bellas was faking it; they had a falling-out. There was talk in the treatment room about an article in the papers written by a close contact of Graeme's that said he was looking to sell Bellas. We were assessing Bellas when the manager appeared and an argument ensued, the upshot of which was Graeme temporarily stopping him from playing. Freddy backed his manager all the way but left the door open to the player to apologise to Graeme and return to the fold. The manager left him out of a couple of matches. That might have been that, but Bellas went on Sky Sports and accused the manager of being a liar. There's no coming back from that. We knew he'd never play under Souness again; they put him out on loan to Celtic.

Alan was out injured at the time. A lot of the fans started questioning Graeme's decision-making in letting a star forward go when we were short of goalscorers. Things settled when we went unbeaten in February and March, including a home win against Liverpool. Before that match Alan was given a special award for scoring his 250th Premier League goal, and then Laurent Robert capped it off with an inch-perfect left-footed free kick from the angle of the box on the right into the top left corner of the goal.

We booked an FA Cup semi-final against Man Utd in Cardiff and were through to the quarter-finals of the UEFA Cup. But then at the beginning of April we went on a run of four losses. The first of those was a 3-0 defeat to Villa at St James'. It was one of those memorable matches in Toon history; first, Steven Taylor got himself sent off (the hilarious exit when he saved on the line with his hand then arched backwards clutching his side and rolled over as if he had been shot). Then Lee Bowyer and Kieron Dyer had their infamous fight and were both sent off. The two lads brought the argument into the dressing room, witnessed by the other sending-off, Tayls. When the rest of the team came into the dressing room, everyone was shouting and bawling. Al bollocked the two lads, because he knew they would miss the semi-final, then Graeme offered to fight the two of them! The event was seen as emblematic of problems within the club.

The injury situation didn't let up. Graeme decided the best way to deal with the large number of injuries was to have them in for three treatment sessions a day: morning, afternoon and evening. That was a problem for us physios. To be able to cope with such a demanding workload we organised for the evening session to be done down at the Riverside ground in Chester-le-Street. This was coordinated with Nigel Kent, the physio from Durham County Cricket Club. Graeme didn't like that. I pointed out that it was impossible to cover every match, home and away, as well as doing three treatment sessions a day. We explained that we knew Nigel very well; he was a very good physio and followed our rehabilitation instructions precisely. That still didn't seem to satisfy Graeme. I could have also said that we had the lowest number of physios for the Premier League and were paid the least. I didn't mention that because it would have been pointless. He told me that he didn't understand why a physio couldn't work *every* day during the season. Don't get me wrong, Graeme is a great guy and in many ways was a very good manager, but his attitude to players' injuries and the subsequent response required from the medical department to deal with them put a lot of pressure on us. The club doctor at the time was Guy Stevenson. It was a difficult time for him as well, but he was always very supportive of the physio staff.

Five days after the Aston Villa bust-up we played Sporting CP at home in the UEFA Cup quarter-final, first leg. Sporting were impressive, but we managed a 1-0 victory when Alan put away one of Laurent Robert's crosses. Lee Bowyer had been put on the bench because of the fight, but when he replaced Kieron they shook hands and were applauded by the supporters. The two of them were good friends and had made up well before that point anyway. What was noticeable was that Laurent wasn't happy at being substituted. It was another one of those periods when player issues seemed to plague the manager. Graeme found Laurent frustrating. He wanted him to do well, starting with him, but would always take him off. To make matters worse, just before the return leg in Portugal, he was quoted in the French newspapers slagging Graeme and the team off. They had an argument on the bus in Lisbon taking us to training the night before the match and Graeme kicked him off!

That match started well, and we took the lead when Kieron raced through like a whippet and put the ball through the keeper's legs. That meant we were 2-0 up on aggregate. They equalised just before half-time, but we were still upbeat because we had the away goal and were still creating chances. On the hour, Kieron pulled his hamstring. They'd been really pushing us, but Kieron was always a threat to them when he had the ball. We missed his influence after he went off. They scored again, but we were still going through on the away-goals rule until Beto headed in with just over ten minutes left. We tried to pull one back, which would have been the winner, but they scored the last of their four goals on the night in the 90th minute. The 4-1 scoreline was no reflection on how close we'd come to going through. That was a massively disappointing outcome: to have played so well for a large portion of the tie, being 2-0 up over two legs then losing Kieron, followed by conceding so late on was hard to take. We had a genuine chance of winning the UEFA Cup that year.

The hamstring injury for Kieron was the start of a season's worth of injury problems for him. He'd been diagnosed with auto-immune hepatitis before the start of 2003/04 and as a result was on varying doses of immunosuppressants and steroids. I recall being impressed by the club doctor at the time, John McKay. Kieron felt there was something wrong with him, but it was the doc who suspected the diagnosis and confirmed it before referring him to a specialist for treatment. Kieron has since been open about his condition (he subsequently required a liver transplant in 2023), but at the time very few people were aware. We weren't sure how he would manage on powerful anti-inflammatory meds. Kieron was desperate to keep playing, that's for sure.

The European match was the Thursday night, then we had a one o'clock kick-off against Man Utd in the FA Cup semi-final only three days later. The lads that were still fit to play were knackered. We had a lot of injuries and suspensions. I remember in Cardiff the bus had to stop on the way into the stadium because of the volume of Newcastle supporters. To be fair to Graeme, he made a point of standing up in the bus and telling the lads what this all meant to the bright-eyed Geordies waving up to us as we inched forwards. Phil Boersma, our rehab coach, travelled down with us, but on the day of the match he failed to attend. We never saw him again; the rumour was that Freddy sacked him.

Regarding the semi-final itself, we were never in it, really. The lads looked weary, soon chasing the game. We lost for the second time in three days by the same scoreline, 4-1. To cap that off, when we were on the tarmac at Cardiff airport waiting to take off, Alan Shearer received a text from Craig Bellamy taking the piss and criticising his performance. Al was raging. He threatened to knock him out next time he saw him. The rest of the season just petered out after that. We ended up 14th. This was when Ferra finally concluded that he could no longer work as a pro football physio. He'd applied to get into Bar school to study to be a barrister, but this course was full-time, so if he got a place he would be away. Fortunately for me, I always loved the role of professional football physio. Although it had some bad moments, in general it was great. Off the pitch, things were going well too. Helen and I moved into an apartment in Jesmond and decided that we wanted to have a family.

* * *

Over the summer, before the new season, Freddy organised to bring in Michael Owen and Albert Luque. Graeme said he wanted

Anelka and Boa Morte but they never came. He did sell Bellas to Blackburn, amid a mini clear-out. One of the other players he brought in was Scott Parker. I think Kevin Keegan was probably the last manager who completely dictated which players did or didn't come to the club, and it now seemed that the directors were the ones deciding the squad. A risky strategy to say the least. A manager should be capable of deciding which players are best suited to the style of play they want to produce.

We started 2005/06 by going out of Europe, losing to Deportivo in the semi-finals of the Intertoto Cup. In the league we started slowly, picking up only one point in the first four outings. The fourth of those was a home defeat to Man Utd. Both Kieron and Emre went off with hamstring injuries. They'd failed our fitness tests that day but Graeme wanted to see how they went. Graeme wasn't happy with the injury situation. We had a theory that the training surface at Darsley Park was at least partially to blame. It had been laid before our return there under Sir Bobby. It was a specially prepared grass surface, but it had a strange feel to it. The soil had a sandy texture. The issue seemed to be at the point of maximum deceleration or acceleration, when the surface had slightly too much 'give' in it. It didn't provide the adequate amount of resistance required. That was our opinion, anyway. We thought it was somehow altering the players' biomechanics. The surface was eventually changed at the request of the club.

In September we started winning, beginning with a 3-0 away success at Blackburn. Alan and Michael were starting to prove to be a very good pairing. Just when it was looking as if we might challenge for the title, Steven Taylor dislocated his shoulder for the third time when we took a risk to rehab him without putting him through surgery. That decision was based on the advice of a consultant orthopaedic surgeon. We would have kept him away from competitive matches longer, but the available fit players weren't considered to be up to his standard. I think Graeme wanted to make a point to the board about lack of depth in the squad. Dean Saunders decided Steven was fit to play when he threw a medicine ball at him in the gym and he caught it without re-dislocating his shoulder. I wasn't so sure, based on our stability assessments. Following a prolonged discussion, we decided to give him a trial run-out away to Liverpool on Boxing Day. I had so much strapping on him that Ray Thompson started doing the robot dance beside him. Sure enough, our worst fears were realised when, within 20 minutes of kick-off and an innocuous challenge, he put it out again. We lost 2-0.

A week later Michael Owen broke his foot away to Spurs on New Year's Eve. We lost that one by the same scoreline. Injuries are part and parcel of football, but we'd had a bad run of them. Albert Luque, Emre and Kieron Dyer had all suffered recurring injuries that season. We decided to move the seniors' training sessions to the academy pitches while we were waiting for the new surface at the training ground to be ready. One of the academy physios, Michael Harding, was having to come up more and more often to give us a hand with the injuries. We soon realised how good he was, so we brought him in full-time with the seniors. He continued to impress and fitted in well with the staff and players. Over the next decade or so he became a reliable colleague and solid friend. At the time of writing, he's now senior physiotherapist at Bournemouth. When Michael moved up, that left Carl Nelson down at the academy, often working single-handed to begin with. Carl is another superb therapist. He's now the academy's head physiotherapist.

We then drew at home to Boro but lost the next three matches in a row. Alan was starting to find it hard at the top level. He'd nearly retired, but Graeme persuaded him to keep going for one more season. He was managing to do it by looking after himself and training hard, but he was starting to struggle a bit with pain and stiffness after matches. The final match of that losing series was away to Man City at the beginning of February. The next day, at the training ground, Tony Toward, the operations manager, brought a letter from Freddy Shepherd for Graeme. The letter told him he was sacked.

At that time, Glenn Roeder was youth development manager, running the academy. He was asked to step up as caretaker manager with Alan as his assistant. Glenn and I went back to the Jack Charlton days, when he was a reliable centre-half. He was helpful the day I arrived, and he was there for another five years before leaving to play for Watford. It was great having him back as manager. He was still the quiet, pleasant and unassuming person that he was as a player. It was nice to have the job security, because Helen was pregnant. We decided to move from Jesmond to a bungalow in Hartford Bridge, just across the road from Hartford Hall where I started my physio career.

We were hoping to get Michael back, but he had ongoing issues with his fractured foot. This was frustrating for all of us. As it happened, he played only about half an hour in the penultimate match of the season. He said his foot still wasn't right; meanwhile the 2006 World Cup in Germany was looming.

Chapter 15

Glenn Roeder

GLENN HAD only been back as the academy director at Newcastle for six months when he was asked to step up. It was a relief that Glenn was in charge, even if it was possibly temporary. I'd learned from the recent experience of other physios around the country that the arrival of a new manager could mean the sack. Although it happened mainly to coaching staff, it did happen to the medical team as well. Glenn was a good friend, so I was happy with the situation. I also knew that he was a skilled coach. He only had a couple of days to prepare before the home match against Portsmouth.

He came in on the Friday and we had a chat before he took the lads. He had a very light-hearted session and concentrated on playing football. There was a change of atmosphere about the place. We all relaxed a bit. Matchday was great. Alan broke Jackie Milburn's goalscoring record, scoring his 201st Newcastle goal to make it a 2-0 win. The crowd and the city relaxed when he took Shola Ameobi's intelligent backheel in his stride and slotted the ball into the bottom right corner of the net.

We then took 13 points out of 15 over the next five outings. During this spell we travelled down to Southampton in the fifth round of the FA Cup and knocked them out with a goal by Kieron in the 68th minute. However, to our despair, his hamstring trouble came back to plague him. We sent him for another MRI scan, but still couldn't get to the source of the problem. We took him down to see a specialist in London. He diagnosed, based on the scans, paratenonitis of the hamstring rather than a tear of the muscle or tendon itself. That would certainly fit with the atypical nature of his injury, as although he would feel it 'go', he was still able to complete matches. It's not likely that a player could finish a match with a tear because it would get progressively worse, not plateau. The specialist assured us that a simple steroid injection inside the affected paratenon of the hamstring, followed by a brief period of rest, should do the trick, and that proved to be the case.

We had a rude awakening when we had a run of three losses in the league and an exit in the sixth round of the FA Cup against Abramovich's Chelsea. However, from the beginning of April, Glenn and the lads pulled it around. A 3-1 win at home to Wigan gave us nine points out of nine. In that match Jimmy Bullard scored a screamer against us after five minutes. Shortly after that, Shola collided with their keeper down at the Gallowgate End. When I got to him, it was clear that he had to come off; his cheekbone was sunken and his teeth were out of place. He wasn't having it; we were 1-0 down and the match had not long started. That's Shola for you. He was always a very brave lad. I told him it wasn't up for negotiation. We got him into the dressing room and when he saw his face in the mirror he nearly died! The press didn't realise the significance of his injury. If it was reported at all, it was to mention an 'issue' with his teeth. The bone holding all his upper teeth had fractured away from his skull! Just a word about Shola. Local lad, of course. As well as being brave, he was very intelligent and such a caring soul. I think he could make a great manager.

Off the back of that win, and talk of getting into Europe, we were next away to the Mackems. Lee Clark was getting a lot of stick from the Sunderland supporters after being spotted wearing the 'Sad Mackem Bastard' T-shirt while a Sunderland player when at Wembley supporting Newcastle. The Black Cats went ahead. Kevin Ball came over to Glenn and did a jig in front of him. They'd clashed as academy managers a few months earlier, so I think there was a bit of history there. Glenn took it in good spirits, but it rightly fired him up for the half-time talk. The lads came out and blew them away in the second half. As Glenn said later, never celebrate until you've won, you just make an arse of yourself otherwise (that last bit's my paraphrase). That turned out to be Alan's last match; not long after he'd scored a penalty, he went down. I went on and had a look at his left knee. It looked like it was a partial tear of his MCL. Alan knew then he wouldn't play in any of the remaining three fixtures, including the final match, which was at home to Chelsea. We won that one 1-0, finishing seventh. That meant another Intertoto Cup place for the following season. Scott Parker deservedly took over the captaincy from Alan.

Freddy offered Glenn the job long-term. I was so pleased for him to get the opportunity. Hats off to Freddy for giving it to him. I wasn't sure if he would. Thursday, 11 May was Alan's testimonial, against Celtic. He was still injured. The ground was packed, reverberating with sound. Black and white and green and white filled the stadium. It was an emotional evening. Even Ant and Dec were there. Some great friends played, including Shay and Harps, Les, Watto, Nash, Rob, Shola. What a wonderful experience. Al had to get that last goal, a penalty of course, in front of the Gallowgate. At one point Lee Clark went down injured. While I was attending to him, he went rummaging about in my bag and pulled out a steak and kidney pie, which he took great pleasure in waving about to the crowd. Very funny. I'm sure he put it there in the first place. Alan Shearer gave all the money he made from the testimonial to local charities.

* * *

This was a World Cup summer, in Germany. Michael Owen had just recovered from his foot fracture, but didn't he have to go and get a serious injury in the World Cup, rupturing his ACL. I watched it happen live on TV. Ferra called me. 'It's his ACL, isn't it?' he said. There was little doubt, and this was confirmed by the scan. That would require surgery and several more months not playing. As soon as Michael was back in the UK I took him over to the Steadman Clinic in the US. We were hoping for immediate repair of his ACL, but Mr Steadman found cartilage damage inside Michael's knee, so he tidied that up and said we would have to wait for that to heal before the ligament repair. So frustrating for us all, but Michael in particular. Regarding the team, Alan had retired, so Glenn needed forwards. He managed to bring in Oba Martins and Antoine Sibierski.

In June, Glenn brought in Kevin Bond as his assistant manager. They'd worked together at West Ham. We started the 2006/07 season early, playing in the Intertoto Cup, but were rewarded by getting through, beating Lillestrøm. In the UEFA Cup first round we beat Tallinn, and in the group stage we beat Fenerbahçe, Palermo and Celta Vigo before finishing with a draw away to Frankfurt; that meant we progressed to the final-32 knockout rounds. This was when the club said goodbye to Ferra. He'd been offered a place at the Bar school, so he was off for that and preparing for the start of the academic year. On the plus side, we persuaded Roddy MacDonald to move back down from Celtic to be Newcastle team doctor once more.

At the end of August my second son Benjamin was born. That was a great time, but very busy. My eldest boy, Jonathan, was a teenager, and I was helping Helen with a new baby! She was a star, though. My job meant I was frequently absent and working long hours, but she never complained about it.

With so many matches coming thick and fast in Europe, we had a slow start in the league, only picking up seven points out of 18. Freddy sacked Kevin Bond when a BBC *Panorama* programme directed mainly at Sam Allardyce alleged that Kevin was prepared to take bungs for players when he was at Portsmouth.

It was at this time I had to do another trip to Vail, Colorado with Michael to get his ACL repair. What a place the Steadman Clinic is. The co-owner was a Texan orthopaedic surgeon called Richard Steadman. He has been described as the greatest-ever sports orthopaedic surgeon. I was there so many times that I became well acquainted with him. He was a lovely man, and very good at his job. There's a corridor in the clinic with photographs, memorabilia and messages from some of the greatest sportsmen and sportswomen that he has treated. He even had one of Buzz Aldrin's spacesuits in his office, a present from the grateful astronaut patient. Other autographs or signed photos were from stars such as Tiger Woods, Dan Marino, Martina Navratilova, Kobe Bryant and … Alan Shearer. Yes, Ferra had taken Alan there in 2000 when he was having issues with patellar tendonitis.

Mr Steadman was so successful clinically that his popularity meant he often had several operating theatres running at once, with his personally selected surgeons performing the operations; he would supervise where necessary. On this visit, Michael's ACL *was* repaired because the knee cartilage had healed; we could finally begin his rehabilitation programme. Michael's rehab started while we were in Vail. Within a couple of days of his surgery we started using the gym at the clinic to introduce some basic exercises while we were waiting to make sure he was fit to fly home. There was an American gentleman who would often be in there when we were. He looked like he was in his late 60s. He was a very friendly type and always made a point of talking to Michael and me. He had some knowledge of the Premier League. I asked one of the other physios in the gym who he was. He said he was George Gillett. The name meant nothing to me, but we were told Mr Gillett owned a large part of the Vail ski resort. He'd also previously been a part-owner of the Miami Dolphins and had owned the Harlem Globetrotters. He was current owner of the ice hockey team, the Montreal Canadiens. *Wow*, we thought. *The guy must be minted.*

We saw him again in the gym the following day. This time we chatted for a while. He told us that he would like to invite us out to dinner in Vail, with Richard Steadman. We were flying home the next day but had nothing planned for that evening, so we gratefully accepted his invitation. However, he said he needed to pick my brains about something related to 'soccer' so he would like to invite me to his lodge in the mountains an hour before dinner to meet his family and chat about plans he had that might involve NUFC. Fair enough, I said. Michael said something about how he might never see me again.

Later that evening a car came to our hotel to take me to George's house. It was a beautiful log cabin located in the Rockies. I met his family; he poured me a drink then went on to explain that he was interested in buying an English Premier League club. He was particularly interested in Liverpool, but he was also considering Newcastle. He asked me to 'sell' the club to him, so that's what I did. I told him about the history, the geography, the people, the passionate fan base. I told him what I knew about the current owners. He was genuinely interested. He particularly liked that it was a one-club city and that a large section of the region followed the team. The hour passed very quickly and we went to dinner in a very expensive Vail restaurant, paid for by Mr Gillett. After Michael and I returned to Newcastle, we thought no more of our evening.

* * *

We played West Ham away in September and managed to come away with a 2-0 victory. Shay had a serious abdominal injury. It was getting towards the end of the match when he went down for a 50:50 ball against Marlon Harewood. He took a blow to the stomach, which is part and parcel of the game. He got back up and seemed okay, but then shortly afterwards collapsed to the ground. When the doc got to him, he was writhing in agony while clutching his abdomen. Shay needed intravenous morphine while he waited for the ambulance. It turned out that he had a perforation to part of his small bowel, requiring emergency surgery. That's a very unusual injury in football. It's likely that Marlon's foot compressed Shay's bowel against his spine, causing the tear. After a few seconds some of the fluid (basically hydrochloric acid from his stomach) would have started leaking into his peritoneal cavity, causing his agony. Fortunately, he made a quick recovery once the surgeons had sorted him out.

Glenn brought in Nigel Pearson to be his assistant manager in October. We had a lot of injuries to deal with, perhaps the most we've ever had, even compared to Graeme's time. Glenn wanted to strengthen the team during the January window, but Russell Cushing bluntly told him that there was no money left. The fans were getting restless. Certain players were being picked out by the fans. I remember they had a go at Jean-Alain Boumsong, who

Graeme had signed from Rangers for £8m not long after he'd gone there on a free transfer.

We picked up a little and managed to get into the top ten, but then had another bad run. The injuries kept coming thick and fast. We were doing our best getting the lads through their injuries then working with the fitness guys to get them back on the pitch. The club had public exchanges with the FA and FIFA about compensation for Michael's ACL injury from the World Cup, threatening legal action. Eventually they were compensated for a significant amount of their losses. The club had been unable to buy some players Glenn wanted in the meantime, though.

A few months had gone by since I was across in Vail with Michael. It was early February 2007. Michael phoned me: 'Hi, Derek.'

'Alright Michael.'

'Do you remember that guy who took us out to dinner in Vail?'

'George?'

'That's him. George Gillett.'

'Aye, what about him?'

'He's bought Liverpool.'

'You what?'

George Gillett and Tom Hicks had bought Liverpool FC for what was thought to be about £435m. I couldn't believe it. I never really expected him to buy any of the clubs. I wonder how close he came to buying Newcastle. Things didn't go too well for the two of them at Liverpool. It's reported that they fell out as things started going wrong at the club. George and his family received death threats. Despite trying to hold on to the club, it was sold in 2010 for about £300m. It's alleged that he's still paying off the debt on the loan he took out. We'll never know how things might have turned out if he'd bought Newcastle. If I ever bump into him again, I'll ask him why he chose Liverpool!

Later in February we knocked out Waregem in the last 32 of the UEFA Cup. We played the first leg in Ghent on 15 February. It was a sloppy match, but Kieron put in a great performance and we went on to win 3-1. We stayed in Belgium that night so it was a good opportunity to see the bright lights of the city. There was a bar directly across the road from the hotel. As soon as we got back from the match, Tommo, Mickey Holland and I headed out. It was pretty dark when we got inside but there was loud music and a fair number of folk inside so we thought we'd have a good time. A few of the guys in there were wearing rainbow sashes. There was a university just down the road so we thought it was some sort of uni do.

Tommo got the first round in. 'There's something not right here, Del,' he said. I thought nothing more of it. One or two lads brushed past us a bit close. *That's funny*, I thought. *It's not that full, so what's their game? Are they looking for trouble?* I knew Mickey and Ray could handle themselves, so I fancied our chances 'in a battle'. It was my turn at the bar. I was served by a bear of a guy with a moustache. Then the penny dropped when I saw him pulling the pint: the hand pull was a giant penis. I looked around; we were in a gay bar. I looked at Ray and Tommo. They were talking to a couple of young guys in rainbow sashes. They didn't seem aware. By the time I got the pints over to them, they were aware. 'Fuckin' gay bar, Wrighty,' Mickey said, laughing. He took a big gulp of his beer. 'Fuck it, I can't be arsed going anywhere else … no pun intended.' We ended up staying to closing time, doing drinking games and getting drunk as skunks with the students. We regretted it in the morning, waiting in the queues to fly home, with heads like beach balls.

At this time Stuart Pearce was appointed as England Under-21s manager part-time; he was still manager of Man City. We talked about me becoming the Under-21s physio if he ever did the job full-time. It would mean a lot of extra work, but of course I was honoured to even discuss it. In March, the Toon went out of the UEFA Cup in the last 16 on the away-goals rule to Louis van Gaal's AZ Alkmaar. That was a lot of European matches we'd played with little to show for it. I remember Tim Krul made his debut for us in Europe and did well. Tim was such a lovely lad, who had that Dutch confidence but was very personable. Come to mention it, Fraser Forster, his fellow academy goalkeeper, was equally as nice. They both went on to be very successful keepers.

Michael finally returned to play in a 1-0 defeat away to Reading at the end of April. We then lost 2-0 at home to Blackburn on Saturday, 5 May. The following day, Freddy Shepherd sacked Glenn (I've written that a few times now!). There was only one match left in the season. One thing about Freddy and the timings of his sackings was that he was predictably unpredictable; two matches in, one match left, in the middle – anything was possible. Nigel was in charge for the final match, which we drew away to Watford. We finished 13th. I really hoped Nige would be given the job full-time. He was no-nonsense but at the same time a lot of fun to be around, an old-fashioned man's man but also with an excellent footballer's and coach's brain.

Over the summer, Sam Allardyce was announced as the new manager. Shortly after that Stuart Pearce took the England Under-21s to the Netherlands for the 2007 UEFA Championship. In the semi-finals the lads went out against the hosts. It was a 1-1 draw after extra time and went to penalties. What made that match famous was that it took 25 spot kicks to separate the two teams!

It was heartbreaking for the boys, but they lost 13-12 on pens. The Dutch went on to win the tournament by beating Serbia. Shortly after that, Stuart was appointed as the Under-21s manager full-time, and he asked me to be the team physio. I jumped at the chance.

Chapter 16

Sam Allardyce

SAM TOOK over from Nigel on 15 May 2007. The chairman had obviously been impressed by his record at Bolton. Freddy told the press that the new manager was bringing in his own medical staff. That was it; I already had my suspicions but that seemed to confirm them. I was pretty sure that I was going to get sacked, along with the doctor, when Sam started. Sam had also said there were things at the training ground that needed attending to. He said we had far too many injuries and he was going to put it right. He had a reputation for the scientific approach, using whatever resources he thought were important to get that vital edge, be that coaching techniques, a scientific approach to fitness, statistical analysis or psychology. I thought all that would be academic to me, because I expected to be swept out as part of his clear-out. At least the fans weren't hostile to his appointment. One or two grumbled about the 'long-ball game' but the majority said to give him a chance. As had been pointed out many times, sometimes a manager must use the long-ball game to suit the team he has but would never consider it with a team of entertainers.

Within a week of Sam taking over, something happened that very few of us were expecting: the club had a new owner – Mike Ashley bought the club. The Halls sold the club to Mike Ashley while Freddy Shepherd was in hospital with pneumonia. Freddy said later that he had no idea it was happening and was subsequently forced to sell his shares. Sir John was always the reluctant saviour of NUFC. I suspect he thought he'd gone far enough, and Douglas wanted a payday. I'm told neither Sir John nor Freddy ever met with Mike. On the other hand, Mike inherited much more debt than he was expecting. Someone couldn't have done due diligence. He installed Chris Mort as chairman. I immediately wondered whether Sam would get moved on without even being in charge for a match. That was no comfort to me because a new manager may well bring in his own medical team anyway. As it turned out, Ashley said he wanted to stick with Sam.

When Sam came in, his medical assistant was Mark Taylor. Mark became Head of Sports Medicine and Science. He'd played professionally in the lower leagues but had struggled through injuries. Under Sam and Mark's structure I was sidelined to work on long-term injured players as instructed by them. I wasn't required for away matches. That was new to me.

I struggled with some of their concepts but, as I did many times in the job, I kept my own counsel. I'm all for using science to enhance the performance of individual players and the team, but you have to constantly guard against letting pseudo-science slip in. I suppose the only way to really guard against that would be to employ a whole army of experts in the various fields related to professional athletes' performances and that would be a monumental task. Will it be the future of football? No doubt it will be for the handful of elite European clubs. The biggest clubs in the world, bankrolled by the wealthiest individuals on the planet will have a complete science department servicing the playing staff.

AC Milan are credited with starting the process through the Milan Lab. I don't think we've reached maximum science yet.

As well as sports physicians, sports scientists, rehab coaches and strength and conditioning coaches, they'll probably use functional medicine physicians. This speciality is developing now. It includes the whole lifestyle of the individual: fluid intake, macronutrient diet, sleep pattern, physiological status, micronutrients and supplementation of diet. Another emerging practice is personalised medicine, which uses an individual's genetic profile to guide decisions on diagnosis, prevention and treatment. Soon enough we'll have personalised *sports medicine* where the coaches are aware of the individual's complete genome and consequently can target training regimes and injury prevention. Come to think of it, future sports physicians for the elite athlete will no doubt encompass the role of functional and personalised medicine in their training.

What Sam and Mark were trying to do was commendable, but they started at the club at the end of the Cameron Hall era. The directors had meant well, being the passionate supporters they were, but most of the money flooding into the game was spent on paying fortunes on players and not so much trickled down to the facilities and staff supporting them. Mike Ashley might have been going to change that, but it was still early days. As part of his package, Sam had been allowed to bring in a large staff with him. On the medical side, as well as Mark, he brought two physios, a Chinese medicine doctor and a promise to access medical specialists as required.

Roddy MacDonald the doc had been head-hunted away from us once again. This time Martin O'Neill took him to Aston Villa. His replacement, Ian McGuinness, was great for me. Ginty was another Glaswegian. He was a good friend of Roddy but was very much a Rangers man to contrast with Roddy's love for Celtic. He was equally competent as a sports physician, though. It was a big help to me having him as part of the set-up.

I remember one of Sam and Mark's theories was that players were picking up muscle injuries because of environmental toxins. I was interested to know what these toxins might have been. Mark said that was what the experts had to find out. I remember the doc having to send blood samples to Northern Ireland for a specialist lab to search for the toxins. I don't think they found any. On another occasion, I took Celestine Babayaro to Paris to have his wisdom teeth removed because he was having too many muscle strains … What a beautiful city Paris is.

My theory with regards to muscle tears is that alcohol plays an important role in some players. Over the years I'd noticed that some of the heavier-drinking lads were prone to muscle tears. That's not to say that all the heavy drinkers had muscle tears and none of the teetotal lads had any. It was just an association. There's a very rare condition called rhabdomyolysis, 'rhabdo'. This happens when the skeletal muscle is so damaged that some of the cells die and break down, releasing myoglobin into the bloodstream. An occasional cause of rhabdomyolysis is a heavy alcohol binge. If it does happen in this extreme form, the result can be catastrophic. My suspicion is that alcohol-induced rhabdo is the extreme form of alcohol damage to muscle, and a much milder form could be a tendency to muscle tears, or strains.

Looking through the literature didn't help; no one else appeared to make the connection. There doesn't seem to be much to back up my hypothesis, but I do suspect in some cases either the muscle cells are slightly weakened or perhaps it's a loss of coordination thing. It could be something as simple as lack of sleep or dehydration. Balance and coordination are extremely complex, requiring good strong muscles coordinating with various nerve impulses and proprioceptor nerves (balance nerves from the joints). Perhaps just a little loss of that perfect mechanism is enough for a muscle to contract inappropriately enough to tear. Who knows? I think that's more likely than toxins, but I could be wrong. A basic study would be fairly easy to do as a starting point.

* * *

To get pre-season training started, Sam took the lads to Austria for a training camp. It was a shock to the system. He tried to inject discipline and had two training sessions and multiple gatherings through the day. One of the activities he had was bike rides in the Alps. We started every morning at 6.30am with a 20-mile ride. One morning I set off with Ray Thompson, Nigel Pearson and Emre Belözoğlu, who was recovering from an injury. There was a lake at the end of the ride. Tommo pushed on with Emre, leaving me and Nigel to catch up. Nige pushed ahead and I was trying to increase my speed going downhill when my front wheel hit a boulder. I flew over the handlebars and went down on the road like a sack of spuds, cracking my head on a rock. I ripped my top and, worse than that, managed to skin half my chest and abdomen as well as cutting my head open. When we got to the lake, I dived in to clean off the blood, tarmac and grit. Tommo tells the story that I wouldn't go in the water until Nigel promised to buy me breakfast in the local café. The tale that I was submerged in the lake up to my neck, whimpering 'sausage and chips please, Nigel' just isn't true. For the rest of the trip I was in agony, bleeding and leaking serum. I had to peel the sheets off every morning. Lovely.

A great thing about that trip was it helped to bond the two halves of the backroom staff, the incumbents and the newcomers. When the trip started, my half felt like outsiders, but as time went by we showed the new guys 'the ropes', and we melded into one team.

Shortly after returning from Austria, we played a pre-season friendly away to Carlisle. Joey Barton, wearing the captain's armband, went down after making a turn. He'd fractured his fifth metatarsal. What a blow. On Mark Taylor's orders, we'd been doing biomechanical assessments on all players. The specialist down in Stoke discovered that one of Joey's legs was slightly shorter than the other. The remedy, or intervention, was deemed to be an insert in his boot. Joey agreed to try the insert out, but he blamed it for the fracture and refused to use them after that.

It was disheartening when Ashley sold Scott Parker and Kieron Dyer to West Ham. Both lads had become part of the city and had a place in the hearts of most fans. They'd been two great pros to have in the team and around the dressing room. It was a business for our owner, though. He made £13m from that deal. Scott was sad to leave the club, but Kieron had reached the end of the road. He'd taken a lot of unjustified abuse from some fans in the latter part of his time with the club and it was getting him down. Kieron had always tried his best and was often brilliant but had been plagued for a while with injuries, although he seemed to be over the worst. Some fans never forgot the incident when he supposedly refused to play for Sir Bobby. The irony was, he always had a great relationship with him. On the plus side, Ashley had just brought in Joey Barton from Man City for £6m, even if he had just broken his foot. Alan Smith came in from Man Utd for a similar fee and we got Mark Viduka on a free transfer. Another plus was that Michael Owen decided to stay with the club.

Sam got the team off to a good start. We picked up 17 points out of 27 and were only one potential victory off fourth place. Joey returned at the end of October but wasn't fully fit. I could see certain movements were painful for him. We then lost two matches, the second of which was a mauling at home to

Portsmouth. Defensively, we were poor in that match. They did enough in the first half then sat back and absorbed our attacks without much threat. They eventually won 4-1 and nearly scored a fifth near the end. It was Sam's first home defeat but the fans who at the start of the season had bitten their tongues and kept quiet were starting to voice their dissatisfaction with the team, manager and new owner. The change was scary.

Before that, Sam seemed to be doing alright but something about the loss enraged a lot of supporters and they started voicing their opinions. Some of the players were shaken by it. From Boxing Day we went on a three-match losing streak. The day after the first of those defeats, against Wigan, Joey Barton battered a 16-year-old boy at 5.30am in Liverpool and was locked up on remand. Joey never makes excuses for himself and he didn't for the assault, but he said later that one of the reasons he had so much to drink that night was that he knew his foot wasn't right and it was depressing him.

Just after New Year we lost 2-0 at home to Man City; the lads played well, but it was one of those matches where our opponents had the breaks and took their chances. It wasn't a good sign when they scored their second with about 15 minutes to go and immediately large numbers of fans stood up and started leaving. There were rumours that Portsmouth manager Harry Redknapp had been tapped up for Sam's job. He seemed to be a popular choice among a lot of supporters. Perhaps some of them were expressing their opinions.

Sam's last match turned out to be a goalless draw away to Stoke in the FA Cup. It was a typical robust affair against a good Championship team, played in the rain. Stoke were well up for it, but our lads rolled their sleeves up and fought out a well-earned draw. I thought if we lost, Sam would be gone. So, it wasn't much of a surprise when we heard three days later that he *had* been sacked. He'd only had half a season in charge. The fans were expecting Harry to take over but when we travelled to Old Trafford on 12 January there were rumours that he'd decided not to come. No one really expected the destruction by Man Utd at Old Trafford, but that's what it was. Nigel was caretaker manager again. It was 0-0 at half-time, but in the second half they tore us apart and towards the end we just couldn't get out of our own half. It was quite a shocking match. Ronaldo scored a hat-trick and they won 6-0. Some of the Toon fans produced banners calling for Alan Shearer to be installed as manager. Instead, they got another hero, my old friend Kevin Keegan.

When I heard Kevin was returning, I was so happy. When I heard Terry Mac would be back as well, I was overjoyed. Mark Taylor, Sam's appointment, was still Head of Sports Medicine and Science. The first thing Kevin said to me was he wanted me at the side of the pitch during training with him and Terry so they could get my opinion on injuries and rehab. They also said they wanted me at all matches and at the front of the dressing room for home matches. We immediately sold an extra 20,000 tickets for the replay against Stoke and the start was delayed while they were getting the fans in. We won 4-1; Stoke didn't have a snowball's chance in hell once Kevin was announced as the new manager.

We were not to get a great run in the FA Cup, going out to Arsenal in the next round. This was the time that Mike Ashley brought in his Continental-style management structure to support both the owner and manager. The Geordies really didn't like that idea at all, accusing them of being the 'cockney mafia'. They had a passionate dislike for Dennis Wise. Kevin insisted he would have the final say in player acquisitions. I wasn't so sure. However, I also knew Kevin. In the past he had a lot to say about player purchases and in fact brought a lot of lads in himself, with Freddy or Sir John signing the chequebook for him. I knew they *must* give him final say, or he would be out the door. Wise brought in Tony Jimenez to scout for up-and-coming players around the world. It was Ashley's plan to buy in young players cheap, develop them at the club then sell them for a profit. The club finished with the services of Peter Kirkley, the head of development who for decades had concentrated on bringing through talented Geordies. The club first noticed Peter when he was coach at Wallsend Boys Club, which was the starting point for many famous Toon careers. Wise thought he was too old. In his autobiography, Joey described Dennis Wise as a 'professional irritant'.

In the league things didn't start so well for Kevin: we went eight matches without a win, only taking three points from a possible 24. One of those matches was away to Villa. A lot of Sam's coaching and medical team were still on the payroll. We went down to a 4-1 defeat. I knew Kevin and Terry weren't happy about the medical side of things. I came in on the Monday morning to discover most of Sam's medical staff had been paid up. Mark Taylor was still there, but before long he left as well. I was then back doing the same job I was doing before Sam arrived. It was a close call, but I was still at the Toon! It was also an opportunity to bring in a physio of our choice, Davie Henderson. Hendo was a friend and Glaswegian colleague of Ginty's (the doc). He'd spent some time on Rangers' books as a player when he was a youngster and was a first-class physio.

* * *

Although Paul Gascoigne left the club many years earlier, we've kept in touch to this day. I've seen him in good times and bad over the years. About this time, he'd been staying in the Malmaison hotel on the quayside. He'd been on a binge of alcohol and other things for a few weeks. His mental state had deteriorated. His sister, Anna-Marie, had been trying her best to get him help, but he was having nothing of it. He wasn't being helped by the guys he was socialising with either. I went into the Malmaison to see him. He was in a right state but refused any help for his mental health; it was his hip that he wanted me to look at. He'd had previous surgery on that. Like Anna-Marie, my concern wasn't really his hip. He was totally paranoid, although he still trusted a random taxi driver enough to send him to the nearest cashpoint with his card to withdraw some money. One of the things he mentioned was his suspicion that his phone was bugged, which of course turned out to be true! The next day he ended up in the Hilton across the river, when things were so bad the police were called to take him to Newcastle General. My brother, John, happened to be the duty A&E consultant and he spoke to Paul and his sister. John organised for a psychiatrist and social worker to attend so that he could be sectioned under the Mental Health Act. I wouldn't have mentioned the episode, but Paul talked about it in a recent documentary.

* * *

Towards the end of February, Wise appointed first-team coach, Chris Hughton. It's probably the best thing he did at the club. Kevin had never worked directly with Chris but had heard great things. Our first victory under Kevin wasn't until we beat Fulham at home towards the end of March. By now Joey had returned after being released on bail and was putting in some solid performances in midfield. We'd been running out of matches to make ourselves safe, but we took ten points from the next four and we were home and dry by then. We eventually ended the season in 12th place. We had a poor goal difference, which reflected some heavy defeats we'd had to Liverpool, Man Utd and Arsenal, but overall not bad, considering the turmoil Kevin inherited. On the downside, Joey was sentenced to six months in prison.

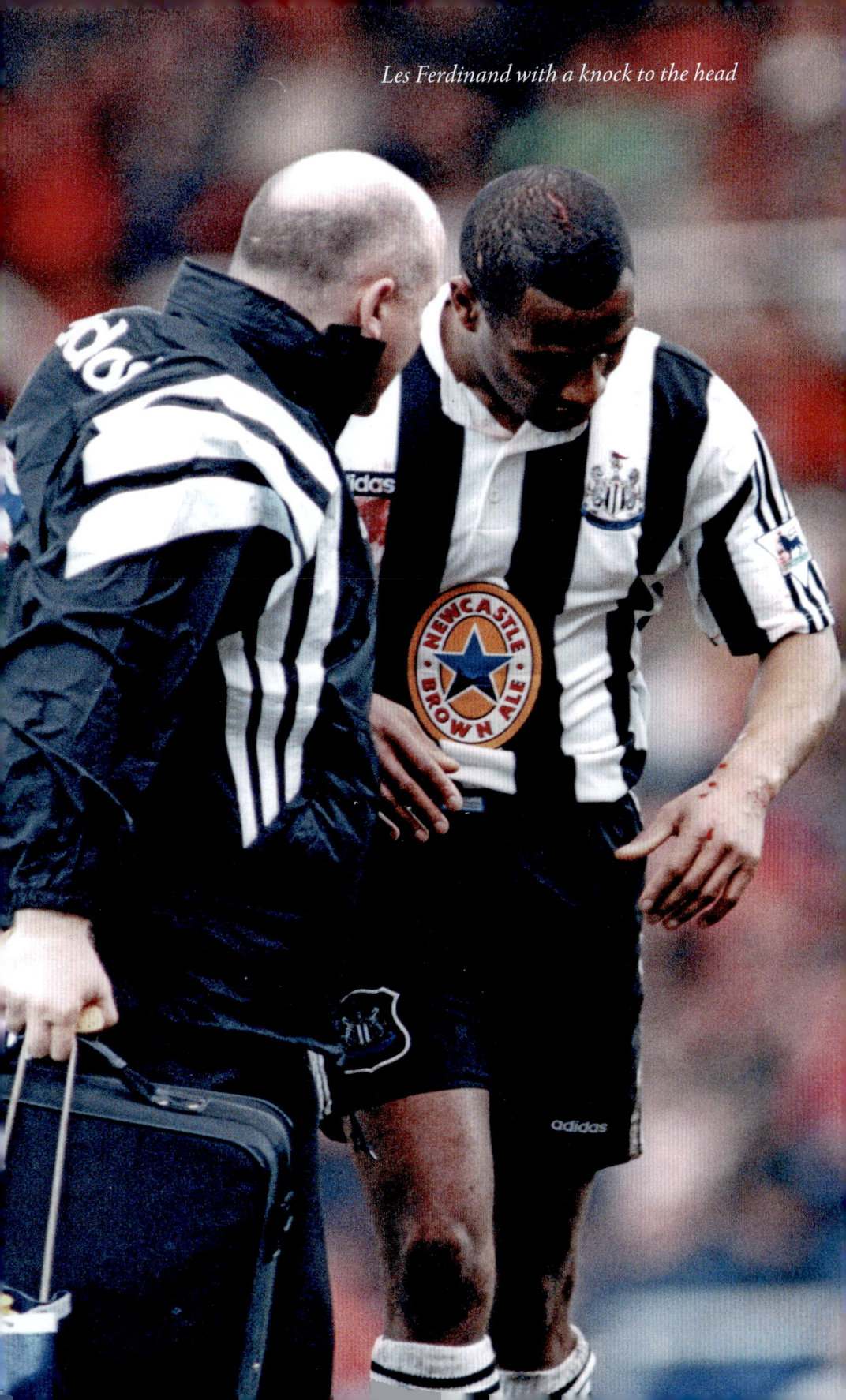

Les Ferdinand with a knock to the head

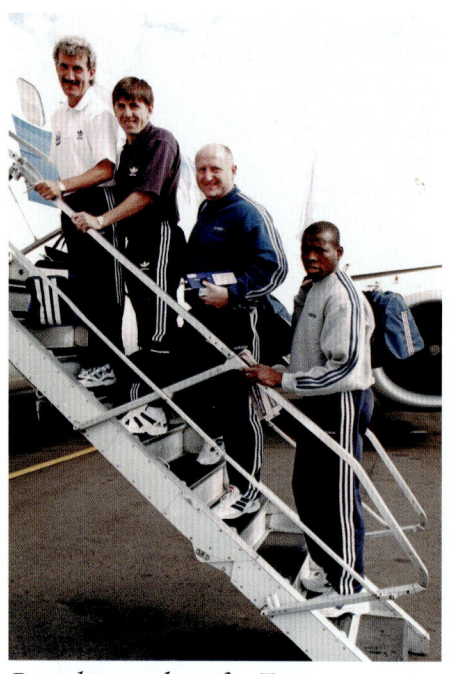

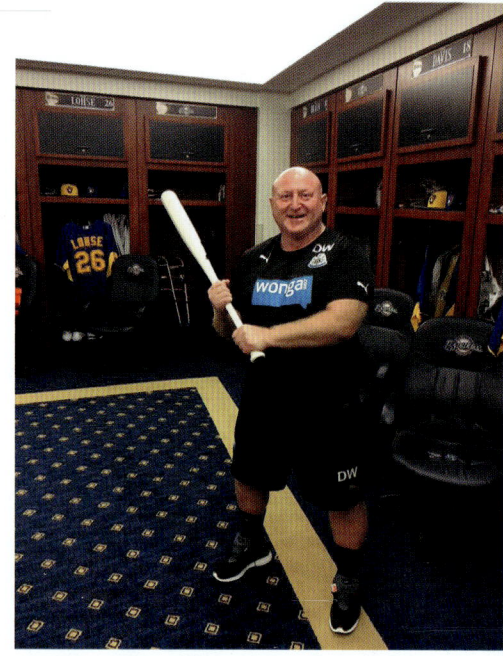

Boarding a plane for Europe. Descending order: Terry McDermott, Peter Beardsley, Faustino Asprilla

Baseball Geordie-style. Milwaukee Brewers' stadium

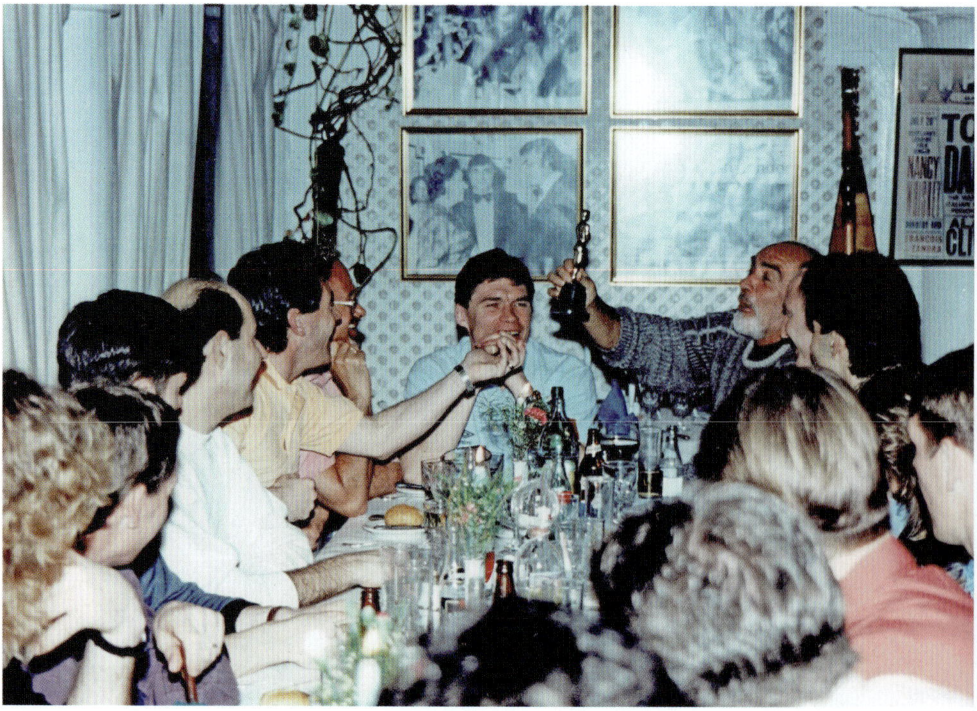

Toni Dalli's restaurant in Marbella. I'm sitting beside Sean Connery!

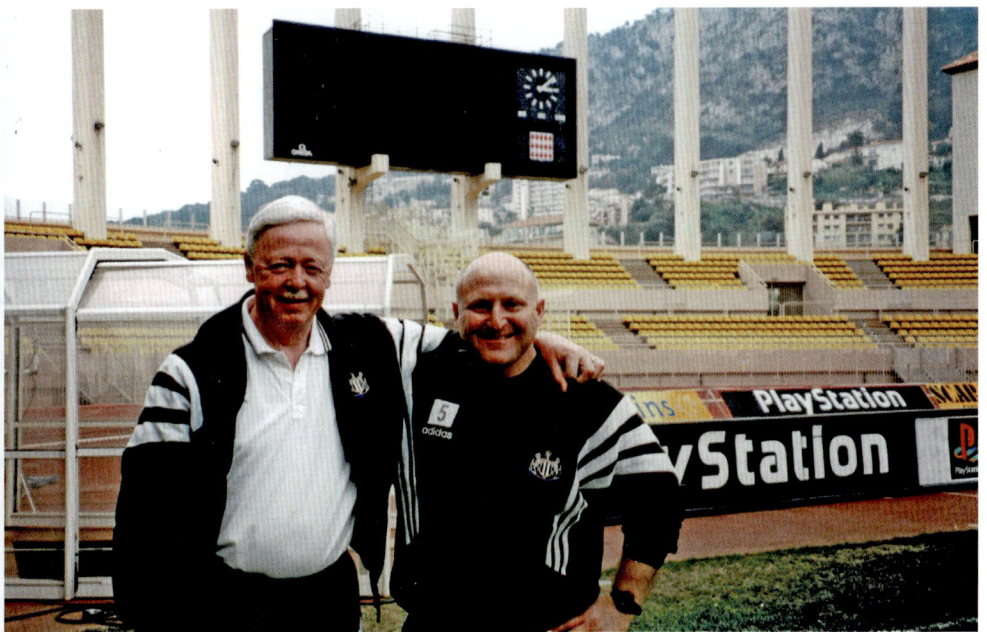

With Dr Keith Beveridge in Monaco

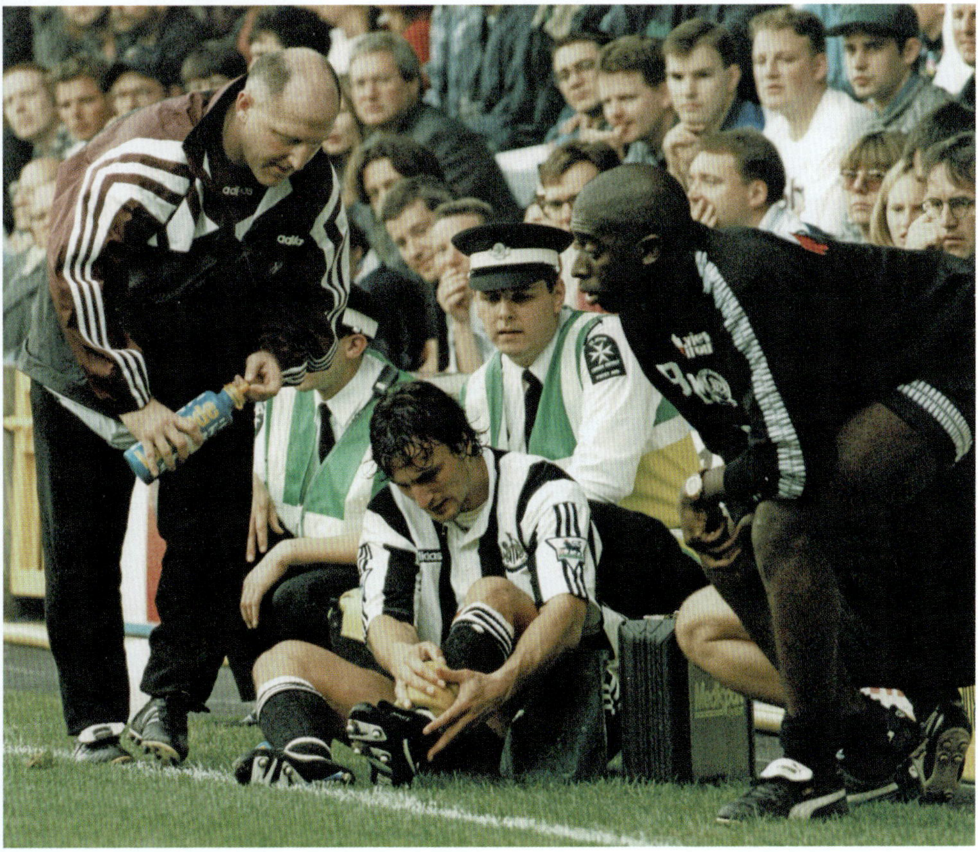

David Ginola injury

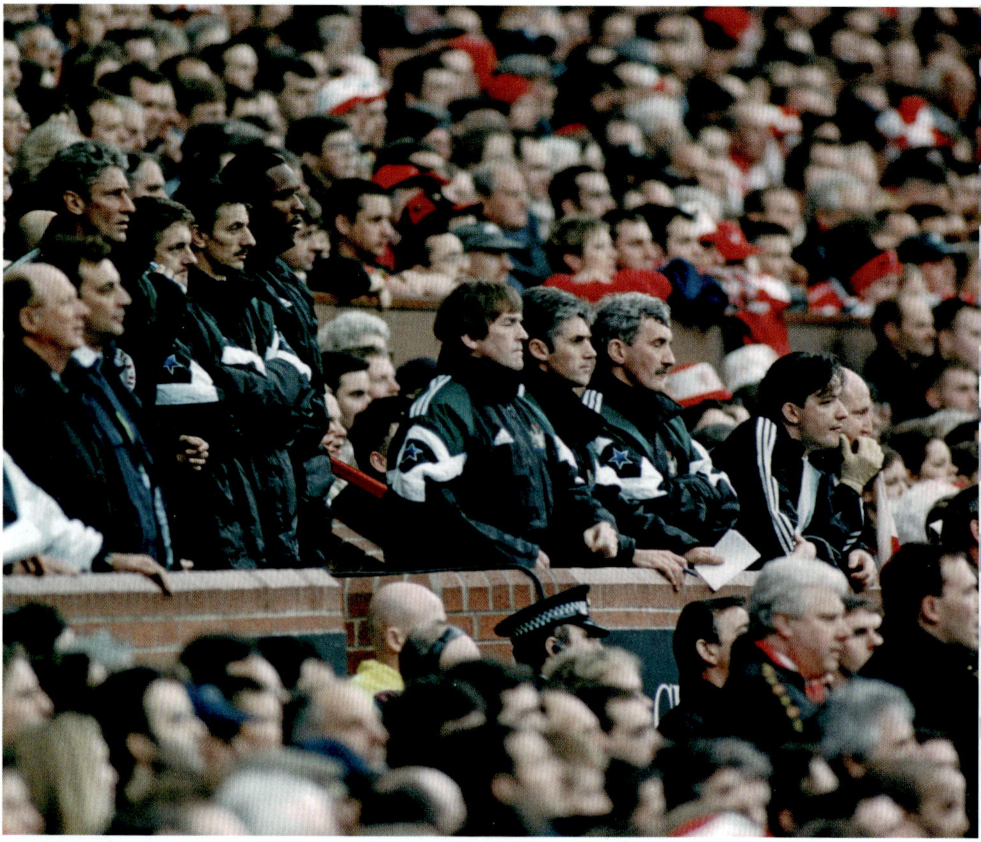

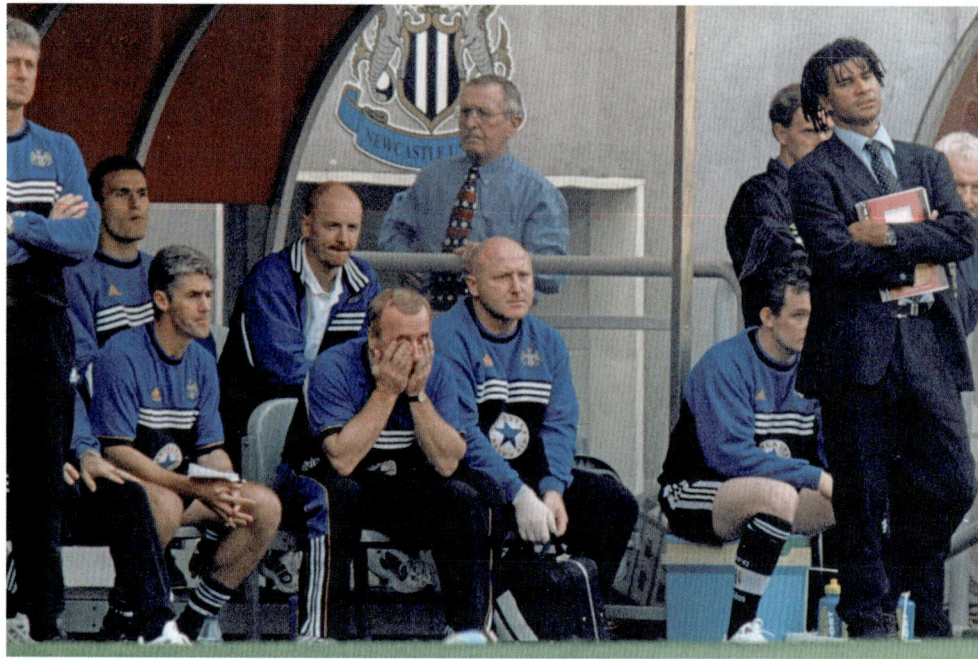

Dalglish bench

Gullit bench. Tommy Craig has his head in his hands

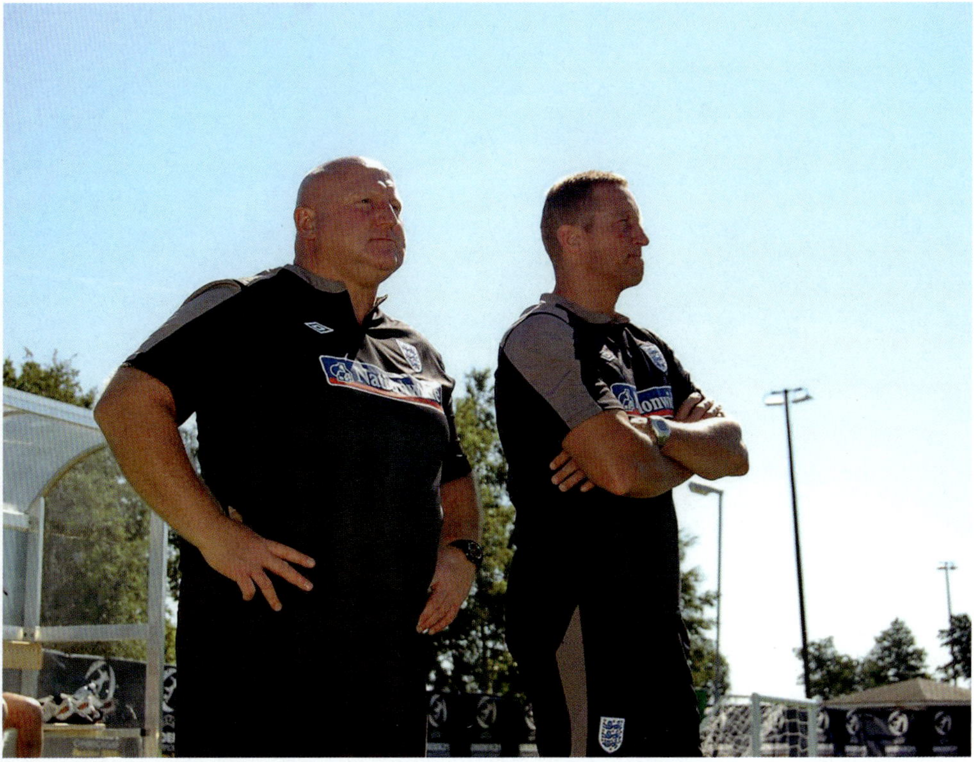

With physio Dave Galley, England Under 21s, Denmark

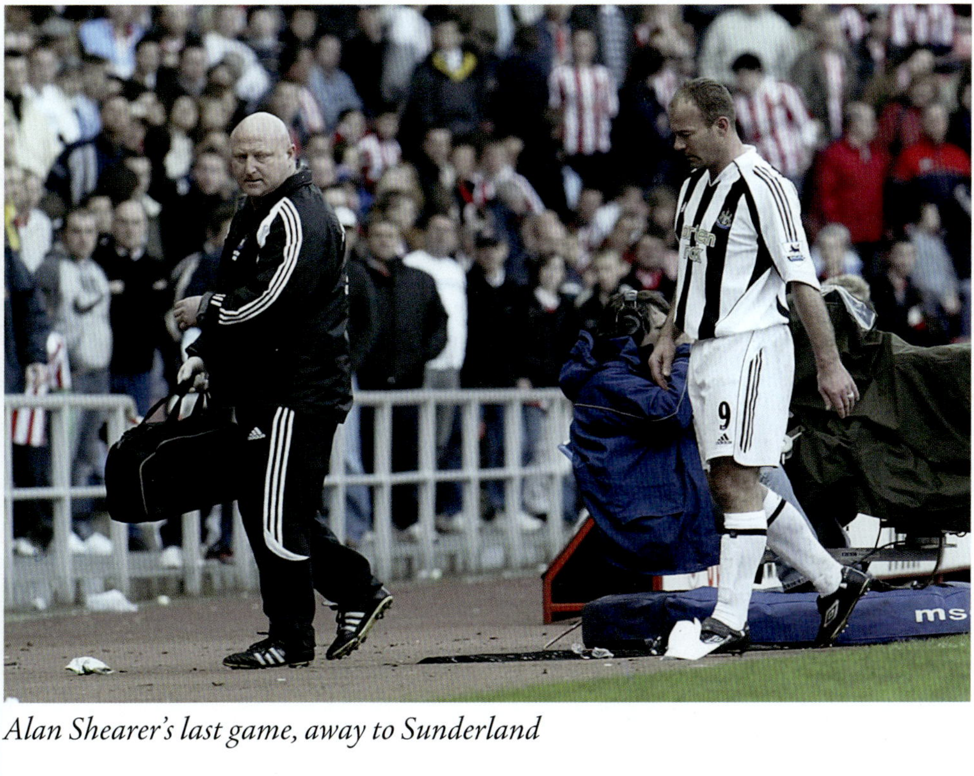

Alan Shearer's last game, away to Sunderland

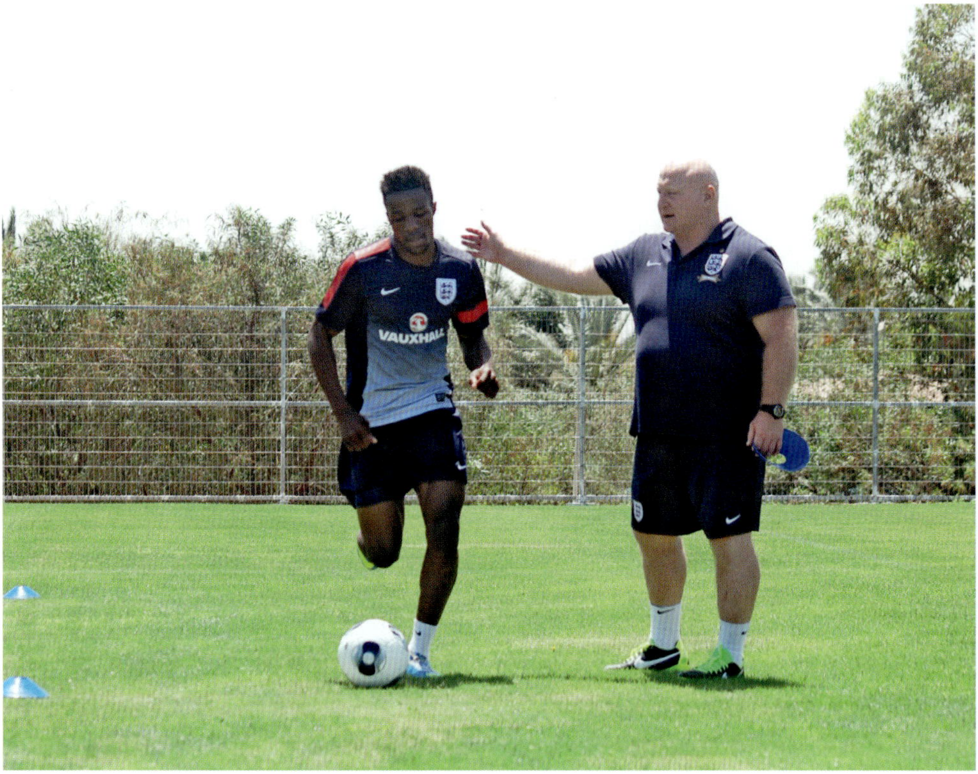

Wilfried Zaha, England Under 21s, Israel

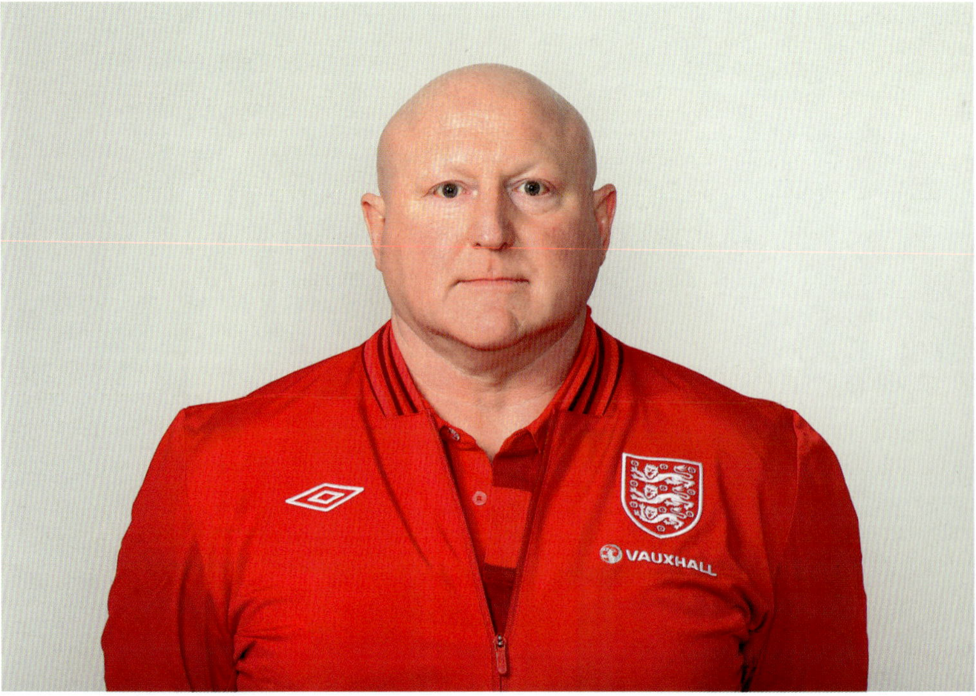

John Bull reporting for England duty

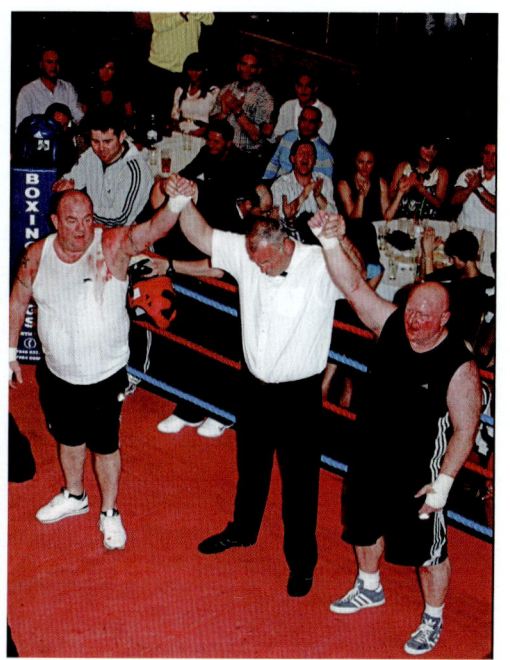

Boxing with Steve Burns (Pugga)

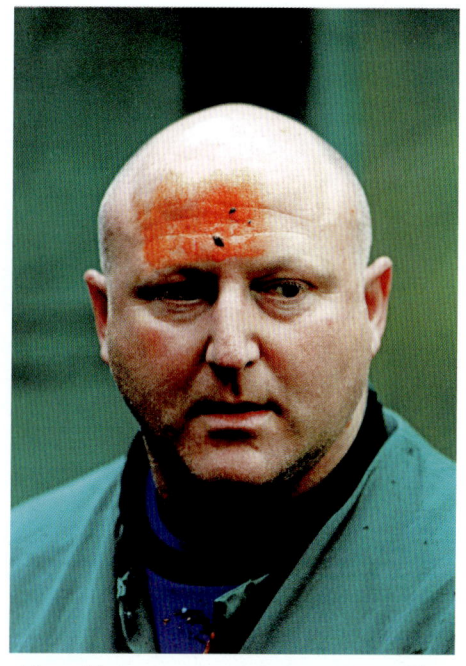

Alan Shearer on target again. We'd just finished paintballing!

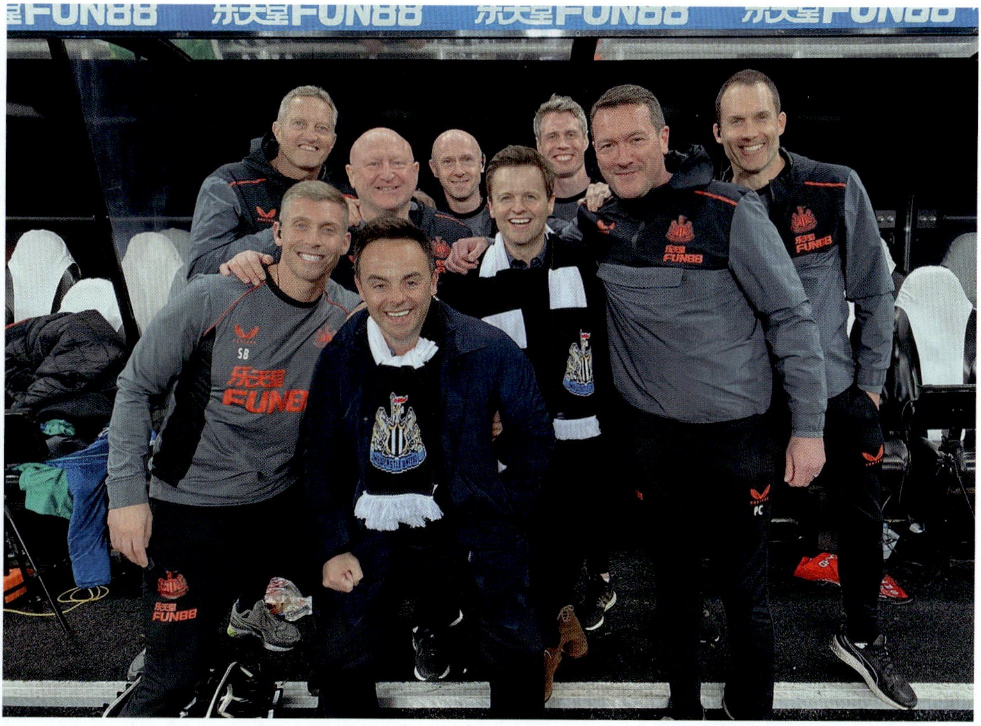

With Ant McPartlin and Declan Donnelly. Sean Beech is on Ant's right and Dr Paul Catterson on Dec's left

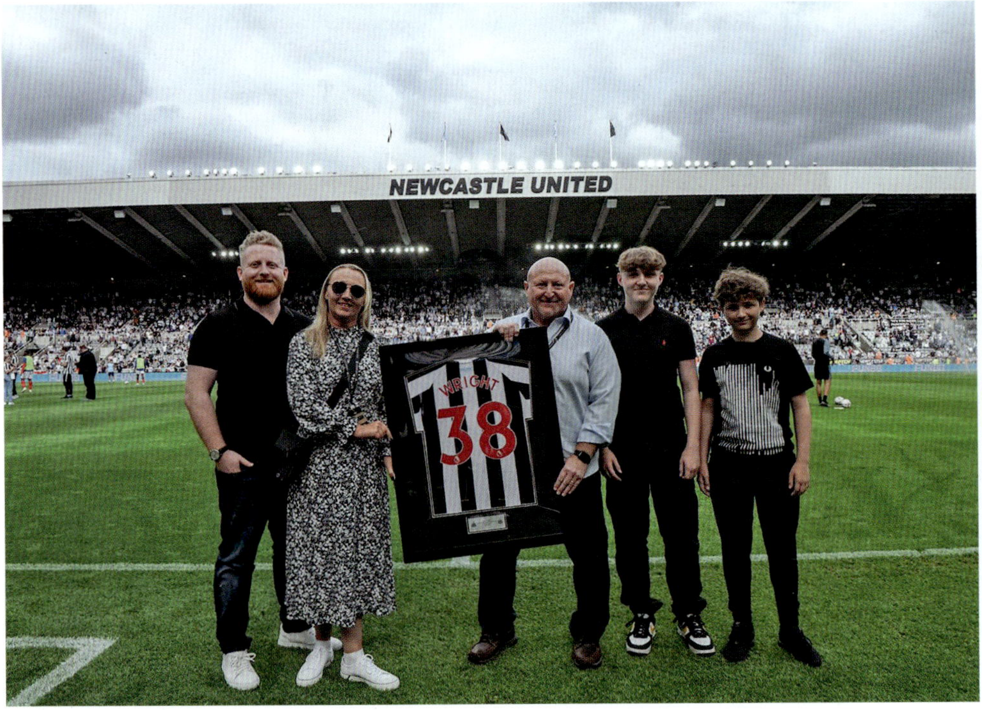

Leaving presentation. Right to left: Jonathan, Helen, Ben and James

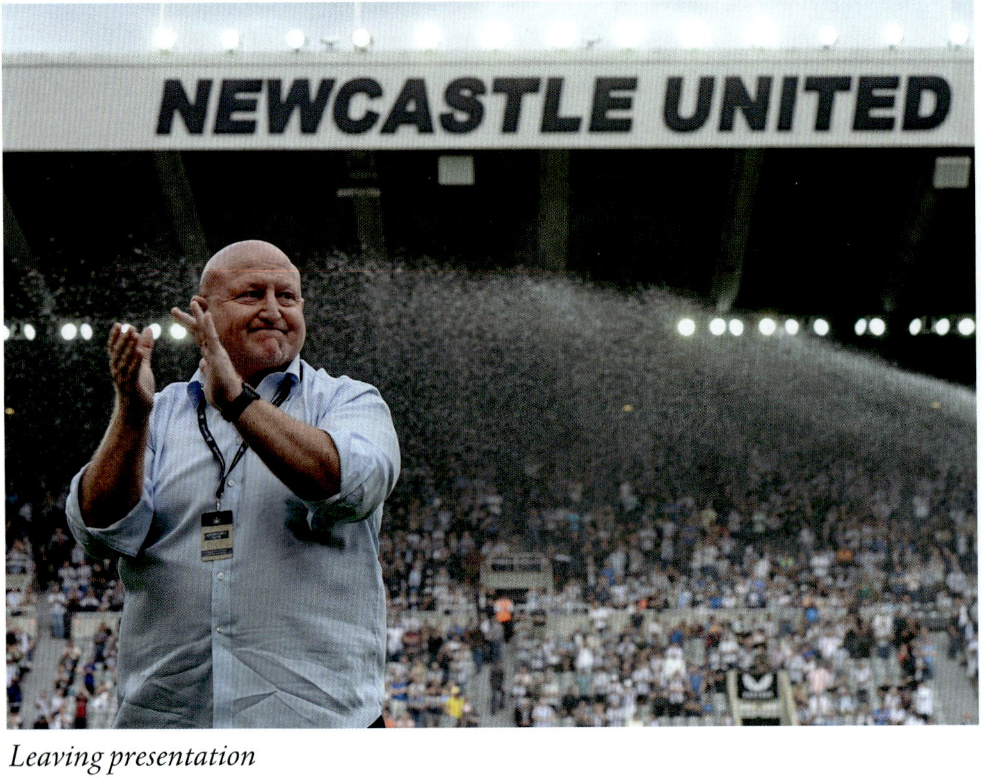

Leaving presentation

Chapter 17

Keegan's Frustration

OVER THE summer, Kevin Keegan had gone on record to say that the quality of our players had fallen a long way behind that of Man Utd. He was frustrated with the lack of communication with the board. I had a good idea what was coming. Kevin is his own man. We in the medical department were always frustrated by the lack of contact from the board. When we did have it, they weren't particularly interested. We weren't the 'sexy' part of the game; that was the team. It's a bit of an incomplete business approach to have but I suspect football is a lot different to most businesses. What always surprised us was when managers told the press how little input *they* had from the board.

Kevin was told through Ashley's management structure that they were buying a couple of new players. Dennis Wise suggested he look them up online. Kevin wasn't impressed. He had an agreement that he would be involved in the final decision about transfers. Kevin phoned Ashley, who confirmed the plans. He then took a phone call from Derek Llambias, who was managing director, to bollock him for talking directly to the owner. Llambias was a former manager of the Fifty Club in London, a private members' club with a bar and casino where he'd met Mike.

The management did sign two guys who proved to be fantastic additions to the squad and would be with the club for several years: Argentines Jonás Gutiérrez, who came from Real Mallorca, and Fabricio Coloccini, who came from Deportivo. Danny Guthrie also came in; he was one that Kevin had found. In the middle of June, my third son, James, was born. Helen continued to be the great mother that she has always been, doing the majority of the 'heavy lifting' required when a new baby arrives. I helped out when I could, one of my contributions being two Newcastle strips for the younger two boys at the first opportunity. I had high hopes that one of them at least would pull on the black and white stripes when they were older. My teenage son Jonathan had started playing for my old team, South Moor Juniors. I gave him the same advice that I'd received: get stuck in, give 100 per cent and don't roll about on the floor if you're injured!

The 2008/09 season started with an away draw at Man Utd. The lads put in a good performance and deserved the point. Kevin was very pleased with the effort. Then we beat Bolton at St James'. We had one or two injuries, so it was nice to pick up the points with a depleted squad. In media interviews Kevin stressed the importance of retaining our best players and bringing in quality to strengthen the squad. He specifically said Mike wanted to keep James Milner even though Villa were reported to be after him. But then James was sold. Just before James went, Kevin said he'd spoken to Mike and he backed up the sale, although he was clearly disappointed.

Next, we went to Arsenal and lost 3-0 in a one-sided match. Kevin had a falling-out with Wise and Llambias because Joey Barton told Kevin and Terry Mac that they were trying to sell him (Joey), which they had no idea about. On the Monday morning Kevin didn't come in for training, although he hadn't officially resigned. However, by the Thursday it was being reported and then confirmed that he'd gone. That was a bleak time, although we were expecting it. No one on the staff had a good word to say for the management structure, but up to that point we at least had Kevin and Terry. As long as they were there, we felt that there was hope of resurrecting the team and making something of the season.

This was one of those low points when all you can do is remain professional and do your job to the best of your ability. Kevin said in a statement afterwards that a club should never force a player on a manager that he doesn't want. Fair enough, you can't really argue with that. It was a huge relief when Chris Hughton was promoted to caretaker manager. Chris was an excellent coach and was always very approachable and supportive.

The home match against Hull was a tough introduction for Chris. There was a demonstration outside the ground and the fans were baying for blood inside the stadium. That was when the 'Cockney Mafia OUT!' banner was unfurled and paraded around the ground. The stewards eventually took the banner, but only after it had gone the whole circuit of the stadium, applauded all the way. The management structure decided to avoid attending that match. No Wise or Ashley to make matters even worse.

Fortunately, Chris was spared the fans' anger. Most people knew he was highly regarded by Kevin. The crowd was able to support the team while voicing their antipathy for the management. We went 2-0 down before pulling one back, but, to cap off an awful day, Danny Guthrie was sent off at the end of the match, which we lost 2-1. The following day Mike announced that he was putting the club up for sale. There was the caveat that if he couldn't sell, he would run the club in a sustainable way. The date was 14 September 2008. We then went on to pick up only two points over the next five matches and lost to Spurs in the League Cup.

Totally unexpectedly, Joe Kinnear was appointed in the middle of this poor run, after the Spurs match and before we played Blackburn. He didn't take over hands-on from Chris until after the loss to Paul Ince's Rovers team. We couldn't believe it. Joe 'fucking' Kinnear seemed to sum up what the supporters had to say. In fact, JFK became his nickname. You would also hear variations on 'Jokin' 'ere' or 'Joke in here'. It wasn't so much about it being him, just that he'd been out of the game for so long. He was criticised so badly by the press when he held his first press conference that it went down in history. He held it at the Darsley Park training ground. The first thing he did was to call one of the reporters a cunt. The next one was told to fuck off. Then he calmed down a bit and called both of them negative bastards. The journalists he picked out had written columns giving him a hard time about not meeting the players on his first day in the job. Welcome to Newcastle, Joe!

At least his first two matches were draws, but then we lost away to the Mackems. The press loved that: it was the first time Newcastle had lost away to Sunderland since 1980 and 19 managers in between. They slaughtered him. One thing's for sure: if you call reporters cunts they'll write negative copies all day long. Joe and the team soldiered on through tough times, but we weren't picking up many points. Then came the 5-1 defeat by Liverpool at St James' Park on 28 December 2008. That was a low point for us all at the club. Shay Given ran straight down the tunnel after the final whistle, visibly upset. He'd played so well, despite the result, and was given the man of the match award. We could tell the award was no consolation to him. A heavy defeat is always hard for a goalkeeper to bear; they accept full responsibility even if they're not to blame.

I still wasn't expecting the bombshell news shortly after: Shay was leaving! We were selling him to Man City. That was a hard one to take. He was another good friend leaving. I'd worked with him under the Liverpool greats (Kev, Kenny, Graeme and Terry Mac) as well as Sir Bobby, among others. He'd become part of the club and city. Other than his goalkeeper buddy, Harps, Shay had been at the club longer than any other player I'd worked with, nearly 12 years. I knew he was finding it a struggle with the changes at the club, but he had family growing up in Newcastle so it must have been a difficult decision to make. Shay played 463 times for the Toon, third in the all-time appearances list, after Frank Hudspeth and Jimmy Lawrence. He was 33 appearances off Jimmy's record, but he'd had enough. Another significant development the day Shay's news broke was that Ashley made it public that he'd decided to *not* sell the club. Just to rub salt in the wounds, Joey broke his foot again.

Not long after Shay left, Joe Kinnear took ill with a heart problem and had to step down. It was the day we were playing away to West Brom. I'd just had my longest conversation with him in the bar the night before. Some days Joe was quite withdrawn and didn't have much to say, but that evening he'd been on good form and showed flashes of why he was so popular with the Wimbledon 'Crazy Gang'. He asked me how many NUFC managers I'd worked for. I said that I thought that he was my 13th full-time manager (there had also been several interim managers that I didn't count) and we joked about that being a bad-luck omen.

He was woken with chest pains later that night, and our doc, Ian McGuiness, suspected a heart attack. He went in as a 999 and required emergency bypass surgery. On reflection from the present and writing this, I know Joe was diagnosed with vascular dementia in 2015. Looking back at videos of Joe's days at Wimbledon, he seemed a very different person back then to the one I knew when he was our manager. I just wonder whether he was starting to have some subtle changes in his personality while he was at our club. It's a shame that I never knew him back in his Wimbledon days, because by all accounts he was a great guy.

Chris stepped up once more. We managed to beat West Brom 3-2. It was a scrappy match but the three points were very welcome. After that, the poor run of form continued and we only picked up two points out of a possible 15. Relegation was looming.

* * *

Then came the pleasant surprise that Alan Shearer was going to take over as interim manager from 1 April. That meant there were eight matches left to stay up. I could see the fairytale script already written down: 'Local hero returns to save the season, then wins long-term contract.' Not only that, but my old marra Ferra was coming back with Alan to be head of the medical department. Paul was at pains to put me at ease. After all, I'd treated him when he was a young player, then was his senior colleague for over 12 years. Paul had formed a close bond with Alan when he was rehabbing his fracture dislocation and I knew he almost went to Southampton with Alan and Iain Dowie.

Could I work with him under the change in circumstances? Of course, I could. We were friends as well as work colleagues. We both do what we do well. Ferra is a good organiser and will do what's necessary to get the job done as quickly and with as little fuss as possible. I was happy to stick with the role of being head physiotherapist. Besides, the first job he did was to ask Michael Owen's individual physiotherapist to leave the building (to be accurate, the club were paying him as a consultant on a pro-rata daily basis to treat Michael). That situation was something I'd been uncomfortable with for months, and Paul had sorted it out in five minutes. As he pointed out, who Ashley decided to pay a consultancy fee to was up to him, but he could work with Michael off the NUFC premises. Alan's team set about changing the dynamics in the training ground, laying down new disciplinary rules and tightening everything up.

The first match was home to Chelsea. There was a sense of anticipation beforehand. Alan received a rapturous reception from the Toon fans, but the team and the fans were subdued by a classy Chelsea team. We were sunk by two second-half goals. Never mind, Alan had just taken over and we thought we had plenty of matches left. Al spoke of a lack of confidence. Next, we were away to Stoke. They were looking to avoid relegation as well, so we knew we were in for a tough match. Stoke took the game to us and went ahead after half an hour. That came from a corner that should have been a goal kick, and when they nearly scored again I was beginning to wonder whether we would come away with nothing. Andy Carroll came on with half an hour to go and immediately flustered their defenders, changing the dynamics of the match. He scored the equaliser with under ten minutes remaining and the away hordes of Toon supporters went crazy. We held on for the draw. That was a promising start.

We only needed two or three wins from the last six matches and we would be alright. What happened after that wasn't for the want of trying. Alan and Iain were usually still in their office after I left for home, and that was a rarity for me to see over the years at the club. Ferra spent a lot of time with me and the doc trying to figure out the quickest routes to return for many of our senior players who were injured. The next match was away to Spurs. Alan went for three central defenders, but by half-time we were 1-0 down and struggling. He managed to get more spirit out of the lads for the second half, but we didn't get any breaks – another defeat. The pressure was on again. After that we were home to

Portsmouth. The fans were up for it, the expectation was a win, no doubt about it. Alan put out an attacking team full of experienced players. Despite that, the importance seemed to weigh heavy on the lads. We never got into a rhythm and any chances we had we didn't take, or David James made one of those reflex saves that he was famous for. A sense of desperation settled around the stadium, and towards the end we were fortunate not to concede when we left gaps pushing forward. It ended goalless; so frustrating. Even one of Alan's teams had to take a few boos at the end when the lads trudged off. We still hadn't won at home in 2009 and we were almost into May. That really was a match we needed to win.

The next one was away to Liverpool. Alan decided to start with Joey. He'd returned from his injury but wasn't fully fit. Every time he put weight through his foot it was painful. Alan wanted to see if he could get through the Liverpool match so he could have an input into the remaining fixtures, in which we had a realistic chance of picking up points. Joey as always was up for giving it a go even though we weren't expected to win; Liverpool were in second place and playing some breathless football during that period.

It was going to script when we were 2-0 down with just over ten minutes left. Joey was still playing, but limping. He'd shown signs of frustration all match. He was suffering from injury and wasn't quite fully fit anyway. He'd done remarkably well to still be on the pitch. Xabi Alonso took the ball down to the corner. Joey slid in. He could have won the tackle, but his foot was high and rolled over the ball. His momentum then took him clattering into Alonso with both feet and took the Spaniard out. It was a straight red. We lost 3-0. In the dressing room after, Alan bollocked him, but Joey went crazy. It looked like Iain was going to have a go, but Mark Viduka stepped in. Alan just let Joey rant and rave. I'm sure

Alan would never have played him again, but Joey had managed to get himself suspended for the rest of the season anyway. On top of that the club fined him £120,000 and told him to stay away from the training ground.

We desperately needed to win the next match, at home to Boro. It was 1-1 at half-time. With 20 minutes to go, Alan took Michael Owen off and put Obafemi Martins on. He scored straight away, which took a lot of tension out of the crowd. We eventually won 3-1. It was our first home win of the year, and we moved out of the relegation places. Remarkably, destiny was back in our own hands. The next match was at home to Fulham. A win should see us safe.

There was a problem with Michael's groin. He could feel something. The MRI scan was normal but that doesn't always mean there isn't a problem. Like all medical tests, you sometimes get false negative tests. Michael made a comment about being out of contract at the end of the season and didn't want to risk it. We had a group discussion with the player. I could tell Ferra was getting annoyed, as was Michael. We decided to wait until the morning of the match but, when we assessed him, Michael still felt something wasn't quite right with his groin, so Alan rested him. We were still confident of the win.

The ground was packed with expectant Toon fans for our final home match. Everyone was full of hope, but the lads didn't start well; they were very nervous, impatient. Fulham weren't playing particularly well either, but they were calm and started stringing together their passes, retaining possession. It was a typically well-organised and confident Roy Hodgson team. The crowd was becoming frustrated. Then disaster struck when they went ahead just before half-time, springing the offside trap. Mark Viduka then netted for us with a near-post header. We thought it was the equaliser, but referee Howard Webb disallowed it. Apparently, Kevin Nolan was the culprit, blocking their keeper. If Newcastle were ever to cite an example in favour of VAR, this incident must be up there in the top five dodgy decisions in NUFC history. Kevin did absolutely *nothing* wrong, but there was ongoing debate about a goal we'd scored against Boro five days earlier involving an obstruction by Kevin, and many considered that was enough to sway the decision. Many years later Howard Webb admitted publicly to Alan that he immediately realised he'd made a mistake by disallowing the goal.

Then double disaster struck when Sebastien Bassong was sent off on the hour. We were chasing the game after that and, although we created chances towards the end, we lost 1-0. A calamity that none of us expected. To make matters worse, Hull picked up a point away to Bolton, meaning we were back in the bottom three and needing more points than Hull in our final match away at Villa.

It was scorching hot for the match at Villa Park on 24 May 2009. The travelling fans were up for it. Plenty of beer on a hot summer's day. The lads needed the win, Villa didn't. Besides, of the four teams that could go down, we'd picked up the most points in recent matches. There were various permutations, but the only one that really mattered was that we needed to get more points than Hull. We were one point behind them with a better goal difference. Andy Carroll was injured, and Michael was still worried about his groin, so started on the bench. It was a scrappy match, neither team gaining control. Close to half an hour in, it filtered through that Man Utd had taken the lead away to Hull. If the result stayed that way, we would only need a draw. The Toon fans picked up the volume. Then, on 38 minutes, Gareth Barry's shot in the glare of the Birmingham sunshine deflected off Damien

Duff and squeezed its way into the bottom right corner past Harp's desperate dive and stretched fingertips.

Michael came on for the last 30 minutes, but his presence made no impression. The team just couldn't get firing. It was gut-wrenching stuff. The clock ticked down. The despair coming from the away Toon support was palpable. Every time I looked over, so many of them had their heads in their hands. Then came the final whistle and that terrible realisation that we were going down. Back in the second tier for the first time since that glorious day back on 9 May 1993 when we beat Leicester 7-1 to escape four seasons in the old First Division.

How different it felt to the last day we were relegated 20 years earlier, losing 2-0 away to Man Utd on 13 May 1989, when we'd known for weeks that we were already down. This was much harder to take. The mind starts playing tricks. It was as if the gods were taunting us. Alan was meant to be the white knight saving the club. Suddenly the timing was all wrong. If we were going to be relegated, why couldn't it have been under Joe? Alan could then step in over summer and make everything right. Life isn't like a redemption movie all the time, sadly. Sometimes it's like a dystopian novel.

The one thing we had to hang on to was that Mike had promised Alan that he would keep him on to start the rebuilding process. I sat in the club van heading back to Newcastle from Birmingham after that match. Tommo was driving and I was sitting up front with Mickey Holland. We didn't say a word for two hours. Mickey suggested we went through all the Championship venues we would be visiting next season and how we would get there. That brainteaser brightened our mood, especially as Alan would be the one in charge taking us there. We were wrong on that one!

The summer recess was my first England Under-21s tournament. I worked alongside Dave Galley, who's a good friend of mine. I'd studied at Pinderfields with Dave years earlier and I recommended him for the Fulham job when I left for Newcastle. The tournament was in Sweden. Stuart Pearce was the boss and he had James Milner, Mark Noble and Joe Hart returning for another tournament. Other notable players with us in Halmstad and Gothenburg were Lee Cattermole, Gabriel Agbonlahor, Theo Walcott, Micah Richards and Jack Rodwell. We topped the group in the first round, beating Finland and Spain and drawing with Germany. We were 3-0 up against Sweden in the semis at one point, but they fought their way back to force extra time. It went to penalties. Stuart's experience was invaluable in focusing the lads and they held their nerve in the shoot-out, winning it. It was our first final since 1984. It was against Germany. They had Mezut Özil playing. We lost some key players through suspension and went down 4-0 in the final. The lads put up a good fight, but we were up against it when they went 2-0 up through Özil just after the start of the second half. They then scored two more in the last ten minutes.

In the world of rugby union, a scandal known as 'bloodgate' began to emerge following a match between Harlequins and Leinster in the Heineken Cup. It was subsequently concluded that Harlequins had used a fake-blood capsule to simulate a bleeding injury to facilitate a substitution that otherwise wouldn't have been allowed. That would have been of some interest to me as a medical professional in sport, but my brother pointed out that the physio involved was Steph Brennan, our Aussie acquaintance from the sports medicine course in Cardiff. Initially, the player involved received a 12-month ban, Steph a two-year ban and Dean Richards, the Harlequin's director of rugby a three-year ban. The doctor involved who, incredibly, incised the inside of the player's cheek in a failed attempt to cover up the deceit, was initially suspended but later allowed to continue practising by the General Medical Council.

Steph seemed to have found himself in a situation beyond his control. The European Rugby Cup appeals committee concluded that the director of rugby had 'central control of everything that happened'. Fortunately for Steph, his ban was later overturned. The reason I bring it up is to highlight that we as health professionals involved in sport are in a different position to coaches in that we must consider medical ethics while making decisions for our players. My experience over four decades in professional football was that we rarely had to debate with coaches whether what we did was ethical. The managers and coaches were always aware of our ethical code as, under most circumstances, it paralleled the ethics that any boss would have to consider. On rare occasions I would have to point out something that might be straying into an ethical dilemma, and, when I did, the manager would always acknowledge that and follow my advice.

I consider myself fortunate that I was never placed in the situation that Steph was. An example of a borderline ethical situation might be a request to inject local anaesthetic somewhere to get a player through an important 90 minutes or so. The problem with that is the lack of pain (through anaesthesia) to a damaged structure could result in permanent damage rather than temporary damage. The risk isn't usually worth taking. This is something that has cropped up, but I've always advised against. If it is to be used, the player must give his informed consent based on the potential consequences, and must never be coerced in any way whatsoever.

Chapter 18

Championship

A PROBLEM with dystopian novels is that the unhappiness just keeps on coming. Alan Shearer, Iain Dowie and Ferra met with Mike Ashley and his team a few days after the relegation. All seemed to be in hand. However, things went quiet from Ashley's end and then one or two leaks got into the press suggesting Alan wasn't going to be the next manager. Next came a friendly away to Orient in July. We put out our first team and they beat us 6-1. Chris Hughton was in charge, Alan and Iain were to have no further involvement with the team. That was another dark day for the club. The lads were ripped apart by Lee Ryder in the *Chronicle*. Words such as woeful, shameful and capitulation were used. He called for an immediate appointment to 'get the mad house in order'. There were a few choice words spoken in the dressing room after the match. The team organised a players' meeting; Joey and Kevin Nolan suggested that those who weren't prepared to fight the club's way out of the Championship should put their hands up so the manager had a team of committed players in the black-and-white shirts. Some said there and then that they wanted to leave. In the press, Ashley was saying once again that he was trying to sell the club and wasn't ready to commit on a new manager at that stage.

That defeat in north-east London wasn't the low point, though. Six days later, Sir Bobby Robson died, on 31 July 2009. He was 76. He'd had bowel cancer in 1992, malignant melanoma in 1995 and tumours in his lung and brain in 2006. He started chemotherapy in 2007 after he'd been told the cancer had spread. Despite that, he'd battled on for another two years, but when we found out, it was still a terrible shock. What a low point, one of the North East's greatest was gone. We knew it was coming. Only a week earlier we attended an England XI versus Germany XI tribute match for him at St James'. That was an emotional day. My son Ben got to speak to Sir Bobby afterwards. Despite being a very sick man, he was as he always was, asking Ben what he was up to, had he enjoyed himself, what team he played for.

In hindsight, those days were a deep trough, but it also marked the start of the recovery for the Toon. We signed no new players but several left. The club released Mark Viduka when the season ended, and he retired. Damien Duff returned to the Premier League with Fulham. Michael Owen went to Man Utd. By the time the season started, there was still no sign of a new manager, so Chris started as interim manager.

We also had a new doctor. Ian McGuiness had left towards the end of Alan's time and ended up in his dream job as Rangers' doctor. We brought in a local emergency physician called Paul Catterson, who had also trained himself up in sports medicine while progressing his way through the registrar programme to be at A&E consultant level. Paul was working down at the academy part-time when he was given his break and asked by Alan to move up to the first team.

We started with a hard-fought draw away to West Brom. Harps went off injured at half-time and Tim Krul came in. He made some great saves in the second half to salvage the point. It was a typical

Championship match: high tempo, hard-fought. We then won the next five in a row. Something had changed; the players were happy and confident, and Kevin Nolan was proving to be a great captain. Joey Barton had played in six of the first eight matches but then had to stop playing to get his foot sorted once and for all. By the time he went for surgery, a fantastic feel-good atmosphere was back in the team.

Chris had a quiet manner about him but was undoubtedly a very good coach and was getting the best out of the lads. No wonder, he was always good fun to be around, while at the same time being honest, hard-working and dignified. Our first defeat was away to Blackpool in September. We got back into winning ways but then had a tricky patch when we drew two and lost two. Chris and the lads steadied the ship when we beat Doncaster at St James'. It was great news when we heard the manager had been given a long-term contract.

By now, Ashley had made it explicit that Alan wasn't welcome back at the club. Chris's appointment was thoroughly deserved. He and the lads rewarded Ashley by winning the next six matches. We had a great Championship team: Andy Carroll, Shola, Danny Guthrie, Kevin Nolan, Harps in goal. Even 'bad lad' Joey was back in the fold, doing his best for the team. Special mention must go for the two Argentine lads, Coloccini and Gutiérrez. Fabricio and Jonás were the heart and soul of the team. Always first in and last out, laughing, joking and singing. Every day they showed, just by being around the other players, how much they loved the city and the team. They were inspirational.

After the turn of the year the great form continued. It became a pleasure to attend training and the matches. The lads were happy, the fans were happy. It looked like we were going to bounce straight back into the Premier League. Sure enough, we knew we'd done it when Kevin Nolan scored two in our win away at Reading, with three matches left to play. We won the Championship with 102 points the following week, away at Plymouth. What a difference a season makes. That was a cue for another celebratory pitch invasion when the travelling Toon army carried some of their heroes, wearing the yellow-and-gold away strips, on their shoulders in a wave of delight.

At the end of the season I stupidly agreed to take part in a 'heavyweight' boxing match on behalf of charity. There were a few of these going on at the time and they were quite popular. Mickey Holland asked me to do it on behalf of 'Mr Newcastle', Steve Wraith's, charity. My opponent was Stevie Burns, or Pugga, the landlord of the Black Bull on Barrack Road right next to St James'. Pugga is well known in Newcastle, with a deserved reputation for being a hard bastard. He was in his early 40s at the time; I was early 50s. I'd never boxed in my life, but I trained for several weeks before the bout. I knew my opponent was competitive as well, so he would be training for it. It didn't help that every now and then Joey would say that he'd bumped into Pugga training in a gym, or passed by in his car, while Stevie Burns was running across the Town Moor wearing a bin bag. It was only after Joey had bumped into him by chance on an incredible number of occasions did I realise he'd made it all up. I was taking whatever advice I could get. Davie Henderson, my physio colleague, thought of himself as a bit of a boxer. Hendo gave me some sage advice, which was to always remain calm. He said the worst thing you could do was to get angry and lose your temper. He also warned me that at our level it's the shock of the pain being inflicted that often leads to defeat.

The bout was held inside the old Fed Brewery premises in Dunston. Stuart Pearce had travelled up specially for it and joined some of the players up on a gantry close to the ring. My 'trainers' were Mickey and Hendo. While I was getting ready and Mickey was tying my gloves on, the ambulance backed up into a bay outside the changing room window. *What the fuck am I doing?* I thought. I remembered my brother, John, the doctor had refused to attend because he thought I was being foolhardy. How right he was. Helen and my dad also refused to come. My eldest boy Jonathan brought a few of his mates. Several of my Greenland and Tanfield mates had made the effort to come too. The contest was three rounds of two minutes. What a piece of piss, I hear you all say. Well, those six minutes are the most physically demanding thing I've ever done. After that night I have the utmost respect for what boxers do. It's such an ordeal.

When we climbed into the ring, everyone went crazy. Before we started, we stood with the referee. I'd forgotten how big Pugga was. He's several inches taller than me. The bell went and we approached each other carefully. We had a couple of gentle parries. I decided to lamp him, but as soon as I opened my guard he landed a great punch in the middle of my face. He broke my nose with his first good punch. The pain flashed through my head and I struggled to see through the tears. *Fuck's sake*, I thought. I couldn't lose in the first round so I knew, whatever happened, I must complete it. I *had* to keep going. Stevie Burns was targeting my nose with every punch at this point. I decided I had to go for it, just to get to the bell, so I let loose. I could hear the lads shouting and screaming. Pugga and I grabbed on to each other for a breather before pushing off and starting again. I heard Hendo screaming something. I looked down to the corner. He was standing there, purple-faced and snarling in his Glasgow accent, 'Fucking kill the bastard, Derek. FUCKING KILL HIM!'

Christ, I thought, *this is the guy who told me to never lose my temper during a fight*. Somehow, I got to the bell. Halfway through the round I was convinced I would pack in at the bell, but I noticed Pugga was knackered. I also saw that he was taken aback that I hadn't folded when he broke my nose, so I decided to keep going. I also had Mickey and Hendo screaming at me to get back out there and pagga him. I don't remember much of the next two rounds other than it was absolute agony, and that Stevie was struggling as well. The end of the bout came. Neither of us had been knocked down. Everyone was clapping and cheering. The result was … a draw. I'm sure I won really, and he's sure he won too, but a tie was a good result at the end of the day. I will never box again. What a mental sport. And to think my granddad, Joe Wright, the miner, was also an amateur bare-knuckle boxer. Not for me. Thanks for the genetic pain tolerance, though, Joe and Dad.

* * *

The 2010/11 season started with our characteristic away defeat to Man Utd, but we then went on to hammer Villa 6-0 at St James'. Andy Carroll scored a hat-trick. We had some strange results after that. We lost at home to Stoke, Blackburn and Blackpool, but on the other hand won away from home at Everton, West Ham and Arsenal. Then we thumped the Mackems 5-1 at home. Chris had obtained the services of Hatem Ben Arfa on loan and signed Cheick Tiote at the start of the season. Cheick was starting to have some impressive performances in midfield. Hatem had looked impressive, too, but he sustained a bad fracture of his tibia and fibula in a horror tackle in early October.

In November and early December we had a run when we only picked up two points out of 15. Despite that, I don't think anyone was expecting the bombshell when Llambias sacked Chris. It was one of those unexpected and devastating decisions. Things had been going well at the club, the lads were cohesive and happy. We were in 11th place. Chris was very professional about his dismissal. What he'd done was remarkable. He'd taken a broken team and resurrected it. He's one of the unsung heroes of the history of Newcastle United. He has one of the highest win records of any Newcastle manager.

What later transpired was there had been a battle between the players and the owner about win bonuses. The owners didn't have a particularly good reward system anyway, but Mike wanted to severely curtail it. The lads quite rightly took issue with that. Unfortunately, Llambias and Ashley had pushed Chris into the fray then blamed him for not sorting it out, throwing him under the bus. To the lads' credit, they refused to buckle to the businessman's pressure to sign what he offered but were determined to do their best, despite the situation. Chris was made a scapegoat and sacked. Some of the players were very angry with that.

Three days later Alan Pardew was announced as the new manager. The feeling among the staff was that his appointment had been arranged well before Chris was sacked and they left it just long enough to look like they'd frantically searched for someone. Pard's installation was another shock. No one expected that he would be announced as manager, not for any reason other than he was not on our, or anybody else's, radar. We looked back at his previous managerial record – nothing there to suggest why Ashley had decided to sack Chris and appoint him. There were rumours that Alan knew Mike from Llambias's old casino, Fifty Club. Didn't really matter at the end of the day. It was another managerial change to survive.

Chapter 19

Alan Pardew Arrives

IT WAS a relief to finally meet Alan, or Pards as he was soon to be known. He seemed a pragmatic English-style manager with no desire to bring in any new medical staff. He assured me that he would defer any decision-making on injuries to us and wouldn't interfere in our day-to-day management of rehabilitation; he was true to his word. He promoted Steve Stone from assistant manager with the reserves to first-team coach. The training sessions were varied and carefully prepared. Pards won over the players with his honesty and obvious ability as a manager and a coach.

We got off to a good start under his supervision, a 3-1 win at home to Liverpool. Before the match there was a fan protest outside the ground. Although Chris Hughton wasn't a particular favourite of the fans to start with, he'd grown on them over time, and many were genuinely upset when they heard he was going. As is usual with most Toon protests while I worked at the club, the fans' anger wasn't directed at the new manager, but at the owner. There certainly was no arguing with the manner of the win over Liverpool, which was eventually comfortable by the time Andy Carroll fired in a long-range shot at the death.

Next we lost at home to Man City. We were 2-0 down after five minutes. The lads played some good attacking football and the fans appreciated that, knowing that the opponents were vying with their Manchester rivals for top spot. After that we had two away matches, a loss followed by a win. At the start of January we took on West Ham at St James' and hammered them 5-0. Joey had a great match for us in midfield. Joey Barton, the guy who many had assumed had no future with us, was playing out of his skin and the fans were loving it. Football can be a funny old game.

The club announced that they were selling Andy Carroll to Liverpool. Andy said he didn't want to leave but Ashley was attracted by the amount of money he could make on the sale. Out of the blue, Pards announced that he was bringing John Carver back to be first-team coach alongside Steve Stone. He now had two fantastic coaches in Steve and JC. Both Geordies, of course. Pards also brought in Andy Woodman, Woody to us, as his goalkeeper coach. They knew each other from their playing days at Crystal Palace, and Pards had used Woody in a coaching role at Charlton. He was a great addition to the staff. He had no idea about Newcastle before he arrived, but he settled in quickly and we all got on together like a house on fire. He raves to this day about what a great city Newcastle is.

There were a couple more additions to the staff at this time. On the medical team, Pardew brought in Wayne Farrage. He introduced us to the Feldenkrais Method, a movement-centred approach to rehab. We had some good results with Wayne's approach and he became an important member of our team. On the coaching side, he brought in fitness coach, Simon Tweddle. Simon was a great colleague over the years. He progressed to become head of sports science before joining Carl Nelson at the academy in that same role.

We went down 1-0 at Craven Cottage against Fulham on 2 February. Shola Ameobi had a clash of heads and suffered the second cheekbone fracture of his career. That injury meant he would be out for weeks, and that irked a lot of supporters because Andy Carroll had just been sold, exposing a lack of depth in the squad. The situation could have deteriorated, but football is unpredictable. Take the match we had only three days after the Fulham one, at home to Arsenal. We were mid-table. We were doing okay in the league, but the jury of Toon fans' opinion was still out with regards to Pards. We shipped early goals; we were three down after ten minutes and four down within half an hour. Some fans started to leave even before half-time but we managed to get to the break without conceding another. I noticed several of the half-time gaps in the crowd never filled after the restart. Joey did what he's good at, and one of their lads lost his rag with him and was sent off. The match was nearly 70 minutes old when we got one back. Within 12 minutes we were back to 3-4. I heard later that some fans who had retired to the Strawberry, Trent House and Black Bull were trying to get back in, unsuccessfully. By this point Arsenal had lost the plot, but we just couldn't get the equaliser. We were entering the 88th minute when Cheick hammered a low drive into the bottom left corner. The stadium erupted in noise. Unbelievable scenes. The ref added on five minutes. The fans were baying for us to get the winner, and Kevin Nolan almost grabbed it, but time slipped away and the ref blew. Never mind, what a result.

Matches like that remind supporters why football must be the greatest sport in the world. Cheick played over 150 times for us and scored only one goal, but what a match to score it in! The 'beautiful game' might not always be aesthetically flawless but sometimes it's wonderfully emotional. It was after this that the fans accepted Pards was their manager and got behind him. He'd skilfully put together a great set of staff and we all got on well together, both at work and socially. He was a good technical coach and a very good man-manager. There was that ongoing rumour that he was Ashley's mate and they met in one of Mike's casinos, but he told us that they'd never met before he was approached for the Newcastle job. He was also thought of as a 'Flash Harry', a bit of an ostentatious cockney spiv. He was undoubtedly always a sharp dresser but the impression that he was Ashley's flamboyant gambling mate never rang true with those who got to know him.

The rest of the season was a mixed bag, but we finished a respectable 12th. During the summer break, Pards bought Yohan Cabaye from Lille, but sold Kevin Nolan to West Ham. I was sad to see Kevin leave. He was an old-school, no-nonsense player and captain and had been a great servant to the club. We were starting to bring in a lot of French players. Many of these were being identified by one of our scouts, Graham Carr. The day after Kevin left for West Ham, Pards brought in Demba Ba, moving the other way from the Hammers.

That summer was another England Under-21 tournament. This one was in Denmark. Notable players in the squad were Jack Rodwell, Tom Cleverley, Kyle Walker, Jordan Henderson, Fabrice Muamba, Chris Smalling and Phil Jones. We drew twice, against Spain and Ukraine, but lost to the Czech Republic. That defeat was enough to see us leave at the group stage. That meant I was able to have a couple of weeks' holiday with the family before going to US with the team for pre-season. While we were away in the States, Cheick told us that he was having problems getting his visa renewed. So, while everyone else was heading home to Newcastle, Cheick and I had to take a detour to West Africa. Although he was from the Ivory Coast, we had to go to its neighbouring country to the east, Ghana. Being a previous British colony, we were told this was the appropriate place to renew his UK work visa.

We arrived at the airport in Accra with our luggage; I was carrying an extra bag containing balls, cones and bibs. I was under orders from Pards and JC to make sure he maintained his fitness for the few days we were there. We were hoping that we would have the visa/work permit sorted within two or three days, if we were lucky. Once we exited the air-conditioned airport, we were met with a blast of heat and, for me, a culture shock. It was a far cry from Ohio, where we'd just been. The place was chaos. We were immediately approached by guys asking to take our bags or to give us a lift into Accra. I noticed three or four guys scooting about on makeshift trolleys because they either couldn't walk or didn't have legs. They pushed their trolleys with one hand while holding out the other for money. Cheick came up beside me and started barking something to the crowds of guys, telling them we needed no help and to back off.

The ubiquitous minivans were everywhere as well, milling about, weaving in between people and luggage trolleys, horns beeping. Out of the melee, a very smart-looking man appeared in a suit. He was holding a piece of card with my name on it. He gave a big smile and introduced himself as George. Tony Toward, our team operations manager, had as usual done his homework and sorted out our hotel and transport. As soon as George appeared, the other taxi drivers melted away. Within 20 minutes or so, George dropped us off at our destination, the Labadi Beach Hotel. This was a great location on the coast. It had a colonial feel to it. They even had a photograph of Queen Elizabeth II behind reception.

Our priority was the visa, so first thing the next morning George met us and took us to the British High Commission (British embassies in Commonwealth countries are called high commissions). We made our way past the security to the area for visa applications. There must have been a hundred people already there. I was the only white person. There was a massive queue. We realised that you had to sit down as you moved along the queue. For some reason, nobody would sit near me, although I was obviously of some interest to them. This was the first of several things Cheick found hilarious. Nobody knew who he was because he wasn't Ghanaian. He didn't speak their language either, but he was able to make himself understood.

'What's up with me, then, Cheick?' I asked.

'They're confused. They can't understand why a white man needs to queue for a UK visa.' He spoke to someone beside him. 'They think me and George are your bodyguards.'

After half an hour or so, we got to the front of the queue. Between the three of us, we explained what we were there for. The member of staff explained to George what Cheick had to do. It wasn't something we could do there and then, so we went off to fill in the paperwork and organise payments, etc. We returned and went through the application process. George told the lady that we needed the visa as soon as possible. She looked at him and laughed, pointing out that the hundreds of other people coming through were saying exactly the same thing. She told us that Cheick should expect to wait two to three weeks for it to be processed. Three weeks! That would mean we missed the opening match of the season at home to Arsenal, and perhaps the next one away to Sunderland. We were asked to move on, so that was that.

As soon as we were outside, I called Tony back home in Newcastle. He said he would do what he could and would let the manager know. Next thing, we had to find somewhere for Cheick to train. George suggested the Armed Forces Sports Complex. We drove there and wandered around until we found someone to ask. They said to wait where we were. Half an hour later word came from the camp commander that we could use the facilities and, if we needed anything, we just had to ask. We found the football pitch. The ground was rock hard and had hardly any grass but it was flat and had goalposts, so we were all set. I put Cheick through a hard training session. Rather him than me, as it was getting close to midday and the sun was blazing down on us. To finish off, Cheick wanted to do some shooting practice. George volunteered to go in goal while I set Cheick up with some passes. Despite still wearing his suit, our driver insisted on doing it. Cheick blasted his shots at the goal while George dived all over the place like a madman. Half an hour later we were done for the day. George was in a mess, but he loved it.

The news wasn't great from Tony. It took him a while, but he eventually got to speak to someone from the embassy. They said there was little that could be done because it was a process that everyone else had to go through. It was also suggested that the player was responsible for the situation. Okay, thanks for stating the obvious. They at least said they would let us know as soon as it was ready. So, we prepared for a long wait. Every morning we went off to the army football pitch and Cheick worked like a Trojan, putting in at least as much work as the players back home would be doing. George refused to wear anything other than his suit, so after every session his lovely white shirt and trousers were covered in soil and grass stains.

On the way back to the hotel each day we passed lots of rickety stalls with locals selling things. Cheick insisted that I try some sugar bread. He said it was a local delicacy. So, we stopped by, and he bought a big packet of it from an old lady. He also bought what appeared to be yoghurt. When we got back to the hotel, George said his goodbyes for the day and we sat down in reception to eat the bread. It was very nice. The rest of the day we chilled by the pool. In the evening, while I was giving Cheick a massage, I felt my guts start to go. Within an hour I was sitting on the toilet and puking into the sink. That continued all night, vomiting and diarrhoea. Hilarious to Cheick, but I was physically unable to walk more than ten yards the following day. George, the taxi driver, took Cheick, the international footballer, training. At one point I thought I had malaria, but Dr Tiote said it wouldn't be that, so I just had to recover from the food poisoning.

I took Cheick training the following day but I still wasn't right, standing hallucinating in the fierce sun, burning the top of my napper, and George jumping round again like a man possessed. It was all very surreal, but after that I recovered. We took a couple of trips to downtown Accra. The markets were something else, lots of hustle and bustle, vibrant colours, music everywhere. Everyone was super-friendly and smiling. Cheick bought me one of those bicycles that the vendors make out of wire and Coca Cola cans. I gave it to my parents, and it still sits on their mantelpiece.

We started getting into a routine, training, wandering about town with George, going out occasionally to bars. Cheick was very easy going; he was a big kid with a big heart really. One thing I noticed when I was doing his nightly massage was that he would get his iPad out and have Skype conversations with women that he knew. I knew he was married, but it wasn't always his wife. He just said he was Muslim and in his culture they were allowed more than one wife. He told me had dozens of brothers and half-brothers because his dad had so many wives. Wow. One of those nights after his massage we popped down to the hotel bar. There looked to be a party going on. Cheick disappeared then came back with company. It was a short, stocky man dressed as a woman; pink wig, lipstick, fake boobs, the works. 'Hi, I'm Princess,' she said in a gruff voice, deeper than Elon Musk's. 'What's yours, honey?'

'Er, Derek. Pleased to meet you, Princess,' I said. Cheick had buggered off somewhere. I managed some small talk for a minute then made my excuses to leave. I was heading to my room when Cheick reappeared with a bottle of beer in his hand for me, creasing himself.

We got past a week, waiting for the visa, and heard nothing. The opening match was getting closer. Tony was making no progress with the embassy, so we headed back down again. We went through the same process, hundreds of people packed in the room, Cheick making out he was my bodyguard, etc. When we got to the window I somehow managed to persuade the clerk that I needed to speak to one of the managers, or whatever they're called. She must have taken pity on me because after half an hour or so I was directed into a room and an English civil servant came in and spoke to me. He said it was impossible to speed things up, but he did promise to let me know as soon as the visa was ready.

The following morning, at the army camp, I received a call from an embassy employee to say the visa was ready. I was straight on to Tony back home, while George drove off to get the visa. Fortunately, there was a flight that night, so we were finally able to leave. We made sure George was rewarded for his first-class service, and Cheick told me how grateful he was for the help I'd given him. I pointed out that he looked after me more than the other way round. We ended up being in Ghana for ten days, but at least we were back just before the Arsenal match. It turned out that Cheick had only missed one pre-season fixture, at home to Fiorentina. Besides, that was abandoned because of rain.

So, we started 2011/12 with a tough home match against Arsenal. Cheick played in a great midfield for us, alongside new signing Yohan Cabaye, Joey and Jonás. I sat with pride watching, observing that Cheick was every bit as sharp and fit as the rest of the players. He ran through walls for the team that day, as he did every match. It ended 0-0. Arsène Wenger seemed more upset than Pards that his team had dropped points, but he never seemed to be happy, so nothing new there. For us, that was the start of an 11-match unbeaten run. It wasn't until 19 November that we lost, going down 3-1 away to Man City, who were destined to win the Premier League that season. By then we'd played 12 times and were in third place.

Then I heard the shattering news that Gary Speed was dead. I was driving at the time. Ian McGuiness, the Rangers doc, called me and told me. I sat by the side of the road in stunned disbelief. I shed some tears; it was a long time before I was able to pull myself together and drive off. Gary had remained a good friend to many of us in Newcastle and it was very difficult to comprehend, especially as he'd been working as normal with Alan the evening before his wife found him. Many of the ex-Toon players would seek us out in the dressing room after a match, and Gary was no exception. I met him a couple of times after he left the club, when he was playing for Bolton. No matter how busy we all were after the match, we managed a quick chat. The last time I saw him was November 2009, when he was on the coaching staff at Sheffield Utd and we played them at Bramall Lane. He came through when I was tidying up and getting ready to get on the bus to head back to Newcastle. We sat for 20 minutes or so and reminisced about the old times. We had a good laugh then went on our way.

* * *

On the pitch, our form dipped for the next five matches, only picking up two points and dropping to seventh. We stopped the rot away to Bolton on Boxing Day. Both sets of fans acknowledged

Speedo at the start of the match. The lads put in a solid performance and had to be patient for the first goal near 70 minutes, but we eventually won 2-0. We then travelled to play Liverpool; Bellas and Andy Carroll were playing for them, managed by Kenny Dalglish. We lost 3-1, not much arguing about the result, but at least we had a great result at the turn of the year at home to Man Utd when we outplayed and outfought Ferguson's team in a 3-0 win. Our second goal was a corker, Yohan hitting a 30-yard free kick into the top left corner. The icing on the cake came when Phil Jones scored through his own goal at the death, trying to head the ball but only managing to bounce it into an empty net.

Nearing the end of the season we went on a good run, winning seven out of eight. One of those was at home to Bolton when Hatem Ben Arfa scored his wonder goal. Just as we were beginning to get nervous, still drawing 0-0 after 70 minutes, Tim Krul rolled the ball to Yohan who passed it up to Hatem, still well within our own half. He made a deft little flick with the inside of his left foot and turned to his right, leaving Ricketts flailing about on his arse. That flick was what got the goal for him, really. After that he went route one straight up the pitch towards the Gallowgate End, outrunning any challenges, and passed it into the bottom left corner. Papiss Cissé scored the second that day.

Cissé was astonishing that season. Pards signed him at the end of January and in the half-season available to him his 13 goals from 12 appearances made him the Toon's most prolific goals-per-game scorer ever. With the season nearly over, he scored twice in our 2-0 away win at Stamford Bridge. His first goal was top class, but the second was unique in its brilliance. He curled his shot with the outside of his right foot. The ball started heading towards the top left corner but, by the time it sailed over the flailing hand of Petr Čech, it nestled in the side netting of the top right corner. The season ended too soon for Papiss, but that goal was quite rightly awarded BBC's Goal of the Season.

We finished in fifth place, our highest in eight years, going back to Sir Bobby's era. It would have been annoying that we'd just missed out on a Champion's League spot, but as it happened Chelsea were able to claim that place anyway because they beat Bayern to win the trophy. That marked Pards's best season for us as manager. The following season we started off having only brought in one player, Vurnon Anita. We had to play a lot of fixtures in the Europa League so, with the flurry of European and domestic matches, some of our star players picked up injuries: Yohan, Fabricio, Cheick and Hatem. Our form in the league suffered and we sank down into a relegation battle. We went down at home to Reading in January and the fans were getting restless. They were also unhappy that Ashley had just sold Demba to Chelsea. He did bring in five new French players, including Moussa Sissoko and Yoan Gouffran. That helped us to start picking up some points in 2013.

On 17 March we were away to Wigan. One of their players made a terrible tackle on Massadio Haïdara in the first half but went unpunished by the referee. JC lost it at the half-time whistle and got himself sent off. They scored the winner in the last minute, which was difficult to take.

* * *

My biggest memory of that day in Wigan was on hearing that Fabrice Muamba had suffered a cardiac arrest in the first half of the FA Cup quarter-final between Bolton and Spurs at White Hart Lane. I knew Fabrice from England Under-21s. It didn't sound good. They said his heart had stopped for 78 minutes. The reassuring thing was that they'd managed to restart it after many attempts at defibrillation. Coming so soon after Gary's death, it was a depressing time. It was great news to find out four days later that he was awake and talking. I was disappointed to hear that he had to retire from the game after that. On the other hand, it could have been much, much worse.

Without knowing the details of Fabrice's medical condition, I can say that professional football clubs today do everything they can to screen out medical conditions that can be associated with cardiac arrests, or sudden cardiac death. All players at the club, whatever their age, are screened by the doctor. This includes a history and examination. The history focuses on any condition the player may have, but also any symptoms that could suggest heart issues, such as palpitations. A family history is also important because some conditions are inherited genetically. Then the player is examined to listen for heart murmurs, as an example. They all have an electrocardiogram (ECG) that's reviewed by a cardiologist. Sports ECGs are a complex subject. After an ECG, they all have an ultrasound of their heart, called an echocardiogram (echo). Again, this is either done by a cardiologist or reported upon by them. One of the main things they're looking for is something called hypertrophic cardiomyopathy (HCM), or sometimes called HOCM. This is a congenital condition that often doesn't manifest until a person dies suddenly (fortunately it's very rare). Most health systems do not have the resources to screen the whole population (the Veneto region around Venice does screen its schoolchildren), but football clubs do. What we've realised is that an athlete could have a normal echo at one stage in their career, but then later can be found to have HOCM. So, what happens now is a player will have a series of echos throughout their time at a club.

Another element to player safety in the modern game is the resuscitation training the medical staff need to undergo. This is done beneath the umbrella of the FA, on the Advanced Trauma Medical Management in Football course. Staff (doctors and physios) must prove that they're competent in first aid, but also basic life support, advanced life support, as well as with orthopaedic trauma management, as a starter. It's not an easy time for us. The course lasts two days, qualification lasts for three years, but a refresher is needed annually. Despite everything, there are occasional medical events that are completely unpredictable. All we can do is minimise the risk to the players.

* * *

In the Europa League we went out to Benfica 4-2 on aggregate in the quarter-final. We were 3-1 down from the first leg when we played them at St James'. Cissé put us ahead halfway through the second half, but we needed that second goal to go through. The lads pushed forward as much as they could and the crowd were fantastic, but Benfica scored an equaliser in injury time. The whole of St James' rose and gave the lads a standing ovation from the pitch.

Three days later the fans weren't so happy when, with a post-Europe hangover, we suffered a 3-0 home defeat to Sunderland, under their new manager, Paolo Di Canio. That was followed by a draw away to West Brom then a shocking 6-0 home defeat to Liverpool a week later. The ground started to empty with half an hour left to go. The last time we lost by that margin at home was 1925 when Blackburn beat us 7-1. We were sinking and just above the relegation zone but a week later fought hard for a goalless draw away to West Ham.

We were running out of matches; relegation was on the cards. The penultimate fixture was away to QPR on Sunday, 12 May. That was a vital match. Realistically, we had to win it. If we lost or drew we knew we would have to beat Arsenal on the final day, and they were hunting for a Champion's League spot. The lads were staying in a posh central London hotel beforehand. We had to deal with all the usual players' issues in the evening, and Mickey Holland the masseur put in a busy shift with some of the lads. We went down to the restaurant and managed to get a couple of beers in and put in our order before they closed for the night.

Mickey must have been feeling flush. 'Fancy sharin' a bottle of wine, Derek?' he asked.

'Aye, why not?' I replied. 'We've worked hard tonight, man. Let's reward worselves.'

'Cloudy Bay?' Mickey asked.

'Sure. It'll cost a bob or two in here, mind.'

'Nivvor mind that, Del Boy.'

I'm not the best at telling stories, so I must explain something about the Geordie accent. In some parts of the region, we love to use strong diphthongs. That is, make two vowel sounds within a syllable. It's so pronounced in some people that the sound ends up as two syllables. For example, Paul, in many parts of the region, is one syllable, like 'call' but with a 'p'. But some people up here make it sound almost like 'Powell'. We also avoid consonants whenever possible as well ... but that's another story. Anyway, in summary, sometimes our accents can be a bit tricky, and people have to interpret what we're saying.

So, Mickey attracted the attention of the head waiter. He spoke to him while cradling his pint, Geordie-style. 'Hiya bud. De ye have Cloudy Bay?'

The waiter looked shocked. 'I assure you, Sir, none of our beer is cloudy!'

Mickey's face was blank. 'Nor, not beeaa ... wine. Ye kna', the New Zealand sauvinyon blonc.'

'Eew,' the waiter replied. 'Cloudy *Bay*. Of course, Sir. Glass or bottle?'

'Mek it a bottle,' Mickey replied.

'Very good, Sir.' The waiter walked off. We were killing ourselves laughing.

'That's worra said, didn't ah?'

'Whey aye, Mickey son, Cloudy Bay.' Or should that be Clewdy Beer?

This is probably a good place to mention some of the great massage therapists (masseurs) that I worked with at the club. These guys are the unsung grafters of the medical staff, using a variety of techniques to release muscle tension and stimulate circulation and range of motion to improve players' performance and reduce the risk of injury. They usually add 'character' to the treatment room. I've just mentioned Mickey Holland who, of course, is also the legendary Batman who crowned Kevin Keegan. He's currently working at West Brom. The first three masseurs we had were Len Clarke, Mick Greener and John Huntley. They worked in the prison service as PE instructors and part-time for the club. Mick was the first to arrive, at the end of Kevin Keegan's first management period. Later we had David Upton, who was with us up until the arrival of Wayne Farrage with Alan Pardew. He's now at Sunderland. Still at the club are Mick Mangan, Barrie Graham and Craig Russell. Craig is on his second spell and Barrie came to us from Newcastle Falcons.

* * *

The following day, after my culturally challenged evening with Mickey, we managed to beat QPR 2-1 to ensure our safety in a hard-fought win, but then lost the final match at home to Arsenal, 1-0. That match, on 19 May 2013, was Harps's last for the Toon, so it was a great opportunity for the fans to show him their appreciation for 20 years at St James'. What a servant to the club. Surprisingly, he made only 157 appearances, but he was loaned out all over the country during his time and, when at St James', was competing with Shay for his place.

During the close season, Joe Kinnear returned as director of football. Most of the fans found it difficult to understand that decision. That summer was another England Under-21 UEFA tournament. This one was in Israel. Jordan Henderson was there for a second tournament, this time as captain. Jonjo Shelvey was also playing, as were Wilfried Zaha and Danny Rose. We lost all three matches and went out. That was to be my last involvement with the Under-21s because Stuart's contract wasn't renewed by the FA.

However, overshadowing the tournament itself for me was the devastating news that my good friend Neil Metcalfe had died. I'd studied remedial gymnastics with Neil at Pinderfields and he'd followed me into pro football physiotherapy. He was at home in Somerset when he collapsed. He was 54. I just didn't understand it. Neil had always looked after himself and maintained his fitness much better than I had.

Chapter 20

Alan Pardew 2

THE 2013/14 season started with a 4-0 loss away to Man City. Arsenal were interested in Yohan Cabaye so he wasn't playing. He also missed the goalless draw against West Ham. We got our first win of the campaign at home to Fulham at the end of August. It was a bit of a struggle for both teams, but when Yohan came on to a mixed reaction from the crowd with half an hour left, he made a difference and Hatem scored the winner after we sustained lots of pressure. He made himself just enough room on the right edge of the box to float a lovely curling shot into the top left corner. There was such a relief throughout the stadium when he scored the winner. To cheer the Toon fans up even more, the transfer window closed, and Yohan was still a Newcastle player.

Steve Harper had his testimonial in September. It was great to see some old faces back at St James'. I managed to catch up with the likes of Sir Les, Andrew Cole and Tino. They were just the same great guys I remembered from when they were players. Alan Shearer and Joey Barton even managed to play in the same team! It was an emotional day for Harps and we were all grateful to be there that day to share it with him. He's a Durham lad, of course, hailing from the pit village of Easington. I formed a close bond with him over the many years he was at the club. He's one of the few players

I worked with who's still on the coaching staff, managing the academy, and that's despite having a brain haemorrhage in 2023!

Not long after the testimonial, Steven Taylor was giving some of us a hard time about our weight. He bet us that we couldn't lose some of it in the next four weeks. As well as me, he had JC, Mickey Holland and Woody the goalkeeper coach roped in. My own target was two stones in four weeks. I had a lot of excess to play with, so thought I would manage it fine. If I lost the bet, I had to run between the goalposts at the training ground, wearing only underpants, while he fired paintballs at me. So what, you say? Well, he also insisted that it was filmed and uploaded to YouTube. My reward would be £1,000.

I made good progress, losing half a stone in a week. The next week I lost four pounds, dropping off the pace, but nothing I couldn't make up. The next week I lost another three pounds. That meant I had to lose a stone (14 pounds) in a week. I kept going and thought I was well on target, but when I weighed myself two days before the weigh-in, I was still 11 pounds off! Steven found out and was cock-a-hoop. I promised him I would do it. He of course thought it was impossible. My motivation wasn't the money, it was my punishment being recorded on social media for eternity. Steve said I would kill myself if I tried to hit it, so I had a word with the sports scientist, Jamie Harley. These lads are all educated in physiology and well-versed in the science of fitness. I explained my predicament, 11 pounds, which is five kilograms to someone like Jamie. He said it was *almost* impossible, but *not impossible*. He also added that Steven might have a point about how risky it was.

I took a scientific approach to it. It was about 36 hours to weigh-in. As a jockey or professional boxer will tell you, at this stage it isn't about burning fat, but about inducing dehydration; that is, losing water. I hadn't eaten that day, so in terms of kilocalories

(calories), just by not eating I would burn 3,000. There are 9,000 kilocalories in a kilogram, so fasting equals well below half a kilogram weight loss. By burning 4,000 to 6,000 calories with exercise, that might get me over a half-kilogram of fat loss. That meant the remaining four-plus kilograms would have to come as water loss. One thing the metric system is useful for is converting weight of water to volume of water. Four kilograms of water is four litres. I knew from my physiology days that would be 40 to 45 litres of water. So, I was looking at a target of at least nine to ten per cent dehydration (to lose over four litres, which equalled four and a bit kilograms).

I called my brother. He said that they would consider admitting someone to hospital with over ten per cent dehydration and give them intravenous fluids if necessary. He added that was nearly always because the person had a medical issue rather than just being stupid, and further added that I should be alright, but it would be a shock to my system. That was okay with me.

When I had the chance to start, I did a HIIT (high intensity interval training) session on the weights, did the treadmill, bike to my limits and went to the sauna. I went back to the gym and did it all again. It helped that I could do some of the workout with Glenn Patterson, the player liaison officer. Glenn is a Falklands veteran and former cop. Furthermore, he's another Stanley lad, from Craghead to be precise. It was a big help having his encouragement. At home that night I had two glasses of wine for the diuretic effect, and the only other fluids I had was sucking on a couple of ice cubes.

On the day of the weigh-in, I got up early, repeated the punishing exercise routine and did the sauna again. I did a sneak preview weigh-in and, unbelievably, I was only a pound off. So that meant a fast run to get a sweat up. By now I was feeling pretty shite but it had to be done. Come the weigh-in, the other three guys passed. But Steven saw me as his winner. I got on the scales and came in just under target! I was paggered, clammin' and parched all at once. Steve couldn't believe it. 'Check the scales,' I said. 'The scales don't lie.' And they didn't. He had Jamie go through all the calibrations but had to concede defeat. Meanwhile, Liz the chef was finishing off cooking bacon and sausages to put into stotties, so I was shouting at Jamie to get a move on. He confirmed the weight. Tayls was gutted. I'd avoided the ignominy of an eternity on YouTube of being the fat bastard paintballed semi-naked. The grand would come in handy too.

Would I do it again? Yes. Was it stupid? Very stupid. No one needs to tell me that. I felt terrible for a week afterwards, with headaches, dizziness and palpitations. So, for the record, it's possible to lose five kilos in under two days but it will not be good for you. Glenn Patterson remained as my gym buddy for the rest of my time at the club as well.

* * *

On the pitch, we struggled in the league but then at the beginning of November we went on a four-match winning run. Next we lost at home to Swansea but then Yohan's goal helped us to defeat Man Utd 1-0 away. It was our first win there since 1972. When we beat Stoke 5-1 at home on Boxing Day, we'd won seven from nine matches. We then only picked up four points out of 24, including a 3-0 home defeat to the Mackems; that run culminated in a 4-0 defeat at home to Spurs. During that period, Yohan was finally sold to PSG. The fans weren't happy, blaming the loss in form on losing such an influential player. Pards didn't play Hatem very much during this phase either. What the fans didn't realise was that the player wasn't seeing eye to eye with the manager.

The team stopped the rot with a 1-0 home win against Villa and followed that with a 4-1 away win at Hull. That was the match when Pards 'headbutted' David Meyler, getting himself sent off. Meyler pushed into the gaffer, who squared up to him with not so much the traditional headbutt, rather the pressing of foreheads. But that was enough to be shown the red card. Things didn't improve on the pitch after that: we won one and lost seven out of eight matches. The final home match was a win, relegating Cardiff, but not much consolation for another disappointing season. There was once again a lot of hostility towards the owner from the fans during that match, and some of that hostility was also directed at Pards. Many walked out on 69 minutes, a time chosen because the club last won a trophy in 1969.

The last match was a frustrating 2-1 defeat away to Liverpool. We were leading into the last half-hour but then lost two goals on dodgy refereeing. Shola was then sent off. It was his last appearance for the Toon, after 14 years at the club, beating Shay's length of stay with us. The travelling fans once again expressed their disquiet during the match. We finished tenth. Alan went on the record to say he needed to bring in new players during the window. Jack Colback came in on a free transfer a week after Ayoze Pérez signed from Tenerife.

* * *

In the close season, I went to Steven Gerrard's villa in Portugal. No, it wasn't a freebie trip, it was work. Ryan Taylor was plagued with injuries throughout his career, not least regarding his time at Newcastle. While with us he suffered an ACL rupture in 2012. We took Ryan down to London for his surgery, but during his rehab he suffered complications because of previous surgery (a medullary nail that had been put in his leg following a fracture to his tibia and fibula had compromised the ACL repair). This was a devastating time for Ryan, but he showed a lot of character and pulled himself round. We took him to Richard Steadman for an opinion on further surgery. Dr Steadman decided to take out the original repair, bone graft the area and then put in a replacement ACL. This meant Ryan being out for a further 9 to 12 months.

Towards the end of Ryan's rehabilitation, Steven Gerrard offered his scouse mate his holiday villa in Portugal. It was a wonderful gesture from him and gratefully received by Ryan. He took me along with him and his family to the beautiful spot. Ryan worked his socks off that week, and we were amazed at the quality of the facilities at Steven's villa. There was a beautiful family home upstairs and games room and spa downstairs, which we converted into a temporary treatment room. The crowning glory of the room was a huge oil painting of Steven Gerrard triumphantly holding up the Champions League trophy.

There was a steam room and sauna included in the spa. We used it one evening before going out to dinner. We had a lovely meal, but when we returned to the villa, Ryan opened the door and we were welcomed by a cloud of steam billowing out the door. We'd left the steam room going full belt! I'm not an art expert and I immediately panicked in case the oil painting had melted. We rushed back and blindly fumbled our way through the tropical dampness to reach the switch. Luckily the painting was saved! With continued hard work, Ryan eventually managed to make his comeback and return to playing. He overcame two huge operations and showed tremendous character.

* * *

A much more serious and painful event happened that summer. Two Newcastle supporters were on a scheduled passenger flight from Amsterdam to Kuala Lumpur. Their names were John Alder and Liam Sweeney; the date was 17 July 2014. They were travelling to the other side of the planet to watch us play in pre-season friendlies against Sydney FC and Wellington Phoenix. When the plane, Malaysia Airlines Flight 17, was over eastern Ukraine, it was shot down. They died along with another 296 passengers and crew. What can you say? Such a tragedy for all involved. I never met Liam, but I had spoken to John on many occasions over the years, usually at pre-season matches in far-flung places around the world. The club did its best to acknowledge the super-fans by opening a memorial garden, flying the flags over the East Stand at half-mast and holding a minute's silence at matches. Sunderland supporters raised over £30,000. It started as a simple floral tribute. As their fundraiser site said: 'There are things more important than any football games.'

* * *

As a group of medical and coaching staff, we were optimistic for the new season. Pards was enthusiastic and continued to foster a great spirit among his staff. We'd had a successful trip Down Under then we'd taken part in a pre-season tournament in Germany, followed by a great night in a bierkeller to celebrate our physio, Hendo's, birthday. However, we didn't make a good start to 2014/15, waiting until our eighth match, in mid-October, for our first win. We missed Cheick, who had been out with a hamstring injury. We were soon in the relegation zone and there was talk once again that the owner was going to sack another manager, so that win gave Pards some breathing space. We then went on to win the next four matches, including an away win at Spurs and a home success against Liverpool. We beat Mourinho's Chelsea at the beginning of December, ending their 23-match unbeaten run. The win was helped by a great defensive display by Fabricio Coloccini supported by Steven Taylor, who was sent off at the death. That put us in seventh place, two points off fourth-placed Man Utd. Pards was awarded the Premier League Manager of the Month award for November 2014, but Tayl's suspension compounded the effects of a large injury list.

The rest of December wasn't good: we lost three in a row, including a home defeat to Sunderland. Both sets of fans came together on 17 minutes and applauded in tribute to the two lads who had died in the MH-17 crash. Adam Johnson scored their winner in the 90th minute. The result was our fourth successive loss to the Mackems, and a section of our home support was very vocal in their criticism of Pards. There were rumours among the staff that he was starting to struggle with some of the abuse he received. However, we managed to beat Everton 3-2 at St James' on 28 December. John Carver did the post-match interview, which raised a few eyebrows, and then the following day we heard that Pards had been linked to the Crystal Palace manager's job. Then the official announcement: he *had* resigned. It was a real disappointment that he was going. Pards and his mate Woody, Steve Stone and JC were a great set of lads to work with but that era had ended.

On Tuesday, 30 December JC was announced as the interim manager. I thought this was his big chance; if he put together some good wins and maintained a reasonable place in the league, he might just get a permanent contract from Ashley. His first match was on New Year's Day, home to Burnley. The lads started well. We were 2-1 up at half-time and playing well. They came into it in the second half and equalised, but when Sissoko scored with ten minutes left we thought we'd won, but they got a heartbreaking equaliser just before the 90 was up.

In January and February we had mixed results, but JC had been announced as the manager until at least the end of the season. Something I didn't want to hear was that Cheick had suffered a knee injury playing for Ivory Coast in the 2015 Africa Cup of Nations at the end of January. On a much happier note, Jonás returned from a loan spell at Norwich to play his first match for the club since cancer surgery. Through March to the beginning of May we went on a run of eight defeats. In one of those, the 1-0 defeat against Man Utd, Jonás got his first run-out. Fabricio handed him the captain's armband when he came on. Two truly amazing servants for this club. We picked up a draw at home to West Brom, then lost away to QPR. It felt like we were in freefall. We went into the final match at home, against West Ham, two points above Hull, who were in the relegation zone.

That was a tense affair, but the fans got right behind the team. It became even more worrying when it was goalless at half-time, but Moussa Sissoko calmed our nerves when he scored just after the start of the second half, and the roof lifted off when Jonás Gutiérrez scored the winner with five minutes left. Everybody knew what he'd gone through. He was such a popular guy, the goal couldn't have been scored by a more fitting person, or in a more fitting match. We'd survived in the Premier League by the skin of our teeth. It didn't help Ashley in the popularity stakes when the club then let Jonás go, and he only found out he was leaving after JC had told Ryan Taylor.

On 10 June, during the preparations for pre-season, the club announced that JC and Steve Stone had been sacked. Steve McClaren was the new boss. He was to be my 18th manager.

Chapter 21

Steve McClaren

SO, ONCE again, a new manager. What was this appointment going to bring? I didn't know Steve. A positive was that he was a northerner. In my mind that meant he was less likely to sack me! I knew he'd made his name as Man Utd coach then manager at Boro, followed by England manager. He'd recently just missed out on getting Derby promoted from the Championship and had then been sacked. He was linked with the Newcastle job before he was sacked, though. The fans were mixed about him. I found him to be a friendly manager. He'd worked with Jim Smith at Derby in the mid-90s after Jim had left the Toon. Pre-season he brought in coaches Paul Simpson and Ian Cathro, and some new players: Georginio Wijnaldum, Aleksandar Mitrović, Florian Thauvin and Chancel Mbemba. Ryan Taylor left for Hull, but thankfully Fabricio extended his contract by a year. What a shame we'd said goodbye to his mate Jonás, who was off to Deportivo.

Pre-season we went off to the US. Andy Woodman was in bits. He told us the story about having his hopes dashed when expecting to get his contact paid up by Lee Charnley, who was the managing director. I've already said that Ashley had finished with JC and Steve Stone when Pards went. This is how it happened: Woody, JC and Stoney had been told to see Lee Charnley at St James' not long before we went to the US. The lads met at the Shark Bar and were having a couple of drinks. JC went up to the ground first, then Steve. They were both sacked and paid up but still had five years of an eight-year contract to work, so were elated. Woody had already been tapped up by Pards to go down to Palace, so he couldn't wait for the five years of salary to see him on his way.

When his turn came to head up to the stadium, Lee told him McLaren loved him and wanted to keep him on! Poor Woody was gutted. Although his son, Freddie, was on the verge of first-team football at Newcastle, he'd decided his time was up and he wanted to move on. He made our lives a misery on tour of the US, bleating on about his contract. On the way out to the States, he told Steve that he thought it was time to go, so at every new city he thought Steve would have a chat with him and tell him he was being released. It never happened. It didn't help that we constantly took the mickey out of him. Just before we returned, Steve put him out of his misery and said he could go. He never got the five years paid up, though, the daft bugger.

Just as Woody was walking out the revolving door of football, an old face reappeared: Steve Black. Blackie, who had made his name with the public as a rugby union strength and conditioning coach, was making a return to the club. We knew him as more of a holistic physical and mental wellbeing coach and that was what Steve was bringing him in for. Steve had worked with Blackie at QPR and Derby and knew how effective he could be. So, it was great to be working again with the ebullient Geordie. He came on the US trip with us. He loved to read and bought so many books when out there that Tommo had to empty half a skip to put them all in to get them back home. I wondered when he would find the time to read them all. Some people seem to live their lives at twice the speed of us mere mortals, and Blackie was one of those characters. It wasn't long before he had stickers stuck all over the training ground with advice on achieving a winning mentality.

We started the season badly, going without a win in the first eight matches and picking up only three points. The last of those eight was a 6-1 defeat away to Man City. We collapsed in the second half. Steve was already under pressure. We got our first win at home to Norwich on 18 October. It was already 3-2 to us by half-time, with Georginio Wijnaldum having scored two, but then he bagged two more as we won 6-2. Then we crashed down to earth, losing away to the Mackems. It was a record sixth consecutive defeat against them. We had our backs to the wall from the moment Fabricio was sent off on the stroke of half-time. It was a soft infringement that lost us a man and gave them a penalty and goal. Before that, we'd dominated. Eventually, we went down 3-0. We were still struggling in December, but managed to beat Liverpool at home, then Spurs away. Ayoze Pérez got the winner in extra time after Rob Elliot had kept us in the match with some fine saves. That got us up to 15th.

* * *

Once again an icy blast to put football into perspective: Pavel Srníček had a cardiac arrest while out jogging on 20 December 2015. We heard he was still alive but in an induced coma in intensive care in Ostrava. There was always hope, especially as Fabrice had pulled through in similar circumstances. Alas, it wasn't to be, and on 29 December, nine days after his cardiac arrest, we heard the terrible news that Pav had died. He was a great friend to many of us, as well as being extremely popular in the city. It was yet another event that was impossible to understand. He was only 47.

* * *

Away from the harsh realities of life, on the pitch we continued to struggle, only picking up two points from the next five matches, although we did sign Jonjo Shelvey and Andros Townsend in January. Ashley had had enough by 11 March 2016, sacking Steve following our 3-1 defeat at home to Bournemouth. It did seem inevitable, as there was constant talk about a replacement and the fans were in open revolt.

Hours after Steve was sacked, Lee Charnley announced that Rafael Benítez was the new manager. What unbelievable news! Rafa's previous job had been Real Madrid's coach. He had an extremely difficult task ahead of him, but the fans loved his warm style in front of the camera. We had staff members who had worked with Rafa at Liverpool. They said he was a good boss to work for, but he was sometimes hard to please and was uncompromising. When I met him, I was apprehensive, but I discovered he was just as pleasant in real life as he came across on TV. He was great at man-management. He also had a lot of clout over the owner, and it didn't take long for him to persuade Ashley to give him more control over signings. Graham Carr, the scout, was sacked at that stage. The manager also brought in a lot of staff, including additional physios, plus fitness coaches, and we said goodbye to many of Steve McClaren's staff, including Blackie. Rafa said he was happy with me remaining as head physio.

* * *

In terms of injury management, Rafa is possibly the most unusual manager I worked for, although I suspect his attitudes and techniques will become increasingly mainstream. Not every manager wants a daily report on injuries, but without fail he would meet with the doctor and me every morning to get an update. We were grateful to have a new addition to the physio team in a fellow countryman of the manager's, Dani Marti.

Rafa was the first manager I worked for who wanted the injured players to start training with the team as soon as possible in some capacity, even if it wasn't the full session they did. What helped in that regard was an additional fitness coach he brought in, Cristian Fernandez. Cristian was specifically a rehabilitation coach. When we were ready, we involved him with the player's rehab. The players would spend more and more time with him and integrate with the fit players as their injury would allow. We would then leave the final stage of return to full fitness with Cristian.

Another unusual approach to training by Rafa was that it was 'light touch'. By that I mean the session didn't last long and he insisted that as soon as it ended the players came back inside. He didn't like them practising free kicks or similar activities once the session had ended. His rationale was that overtraining led to injuries. To help him with this was his head fitness coach, Francisco de Miguel Moreno. Paco was extremely knowledgeable in the science of athletic performance. Modern IT allows rapid assimilation of huge amounts of data that can be easily carried on electronic devices by coaches. All aspects of the players' athletic performance were monitored, such as strength, agility, aerobic and anaerobic capacity. Everything was captured in data form in one way or another and found its way on to his databases. Once he had his baselines, he was able to follow the players through the season and tailor sessions on both a group and individual basis.

Jamie Harley was our sports scientist before Rafa arrived. His philosophy on training was like that of Paco and Rafa, so they worked well together. I'm not an exercise physiologist, but the 'light touch' rationale goes something like this: we tend to think that athletic growth/improvement of any type is linear; for example, put in an ounce of effort and get out an ounce of reward, be that muscle gain, aerobic fitness or weight loss. However, growth is rarely linear like that. The good news is that most growth in human performance is logarithmic. That means with relatively little effort, the early rewards are high. But there's a point reached when any further improvement requires increased effort; that is, diminishing returns for increased work. As the effort increases to achieve maximum fitness, the likelihood of negative effects increases, be that fatigue, psychological distress or injury. The other piece of good news is that the likelihood of injury is neither linear nor logarithmic, but exponential. That means a lot of effort can be put in without increasing the risk of injury rate much, but at some point any further increase in effort *dramatically* increases the risk of injury.

I've heard it said that for professional footballers, approximately 90 per cent of maximum fitness is what the target should be. This 'sweet spot' is what Jamie, Paco and Rafa aimed for, but they did so in a way that they could use objective measurements to confirm. If the player was at the desired level, they didn't increase effort further and therefore avoided the risky part of the exponential training curve with regards to injuries. One or two players even complained that they weren't training hard enough, but the science guys were able to demonstrate to them using their data on the laptop that they were indeed fit enough. Did it work? Emphatically yes, as we had a significant decrease in our injuries under Rafa.

* * *

Rafa's first match in charge was away to Leicester. We lost, but our opponents went on to be champions that season. The travelling Toon supporters took heart that they could see improved performances from the players. The problem was that we were second from bottom with only nine matches to go. It took a while to get started, taking only one point from the next three matches. The first of those was a 1-1 home draw against Sunderland. It was looking dire when we lost away to Norwich, as they were six points above us but had played one match more. We then lost away to Southampton. We didn't play well at all, but our travelling supporters were great and applauded the lads off the pitch. That impressed Rafa no end. After the match at St Mary's, Sunderland were just above us in the relegation zone, two points ahead but having played one match fewer. We were also ten adrift of them in goal difference.

It had to happen, and Rafa's magic finally started to work; we went on a six-match unbeaten run, but there were three draws in that run. It was the last of those draws, away to relegated Villa, that was effectively enough to see us go down when Sunderland beat Chelsea 3-2 at home, leaving them one point ahead of us with a match in hand. They sealed our fate when they beat Everton at home in midweek: we couldn't catch them. Our final match was at home to Spurs. We were 2-1 ahead on 67 minutes when Alek Mitrović was sent off. Spurs were pushing for runners-up spot. Despite being down to ten men we went on to win 5-1. The supporters were in fine fettle, hoping that the gloom of being in the lower tier would be tempered by having Rafa in charge, *if* he wanted to stay.

Nevertheless, despite a great ending to the season, we were back in the Championship. The Toon have been relegated six times in their history and this was the third time in my career. The Mackems hired a plane to fly over the stadium, bidding us farewell to the Premier League. The banner read, '*AUF WIEDERSEHEN PREM TYNE TO GO.*'

Chapter 22

Rafa Benítez

RAFA REWARDED the warm support he received from the fans and the city by deciding to stay, even though we'd been relegated and he had a clause in his contract that he could have used to leave. He'd also received offers to go elsewhere.

In the close season he moved on a lot of the lads and brought in players who could withstand the pressures of the Championship to get us out, such as Matt Ritchie and Ciaran Clark. Rafa also managed to retain Ayoze Pérez and brought in Christian Atsu on loan.

We had a real shock to the start of the season, losing the first two matches. Rafa steadied the ship, and we went on to win the next five. Winning became a habit again. This season was typical of my experience of the Championship, winning lots of matches with a group of players who are committed to fighting for the club and city. The fans were loving it too. We went to Elland Road towards the end of November on a high. Both sets of fans had a great tribute to Speedo on the fifth anniversary of his death. Other than that, their fans did their best to unsettle the lads, but we put in another solid display and Dwight Gayle got both goals in our 2-0 win. We dropped some more points after that, but we never went long without a win.

Cheick Tiote had been struggling to get his place under Rafa and he broke the news to me one day at the end of January that it looked like he was leaving to play in China. He could see my genuine disappointment that he was leaving after nearly seven years at the club. 'Don't, worry, Derek,' he said. 'We'll always have Ghana.'

'Aye, that we will,' I replied, shaking his hand. A couple of days later he'd gone.

* * *

The lads kept up the wins throughout the rest of 2017. We had the opportunity to confirm our immediate return to the Premier League at home to Preston. Christian Atsu scored on half-time to put us 2-1 up. Ayo and Matt added another two in the second half to make it 4-1. That sparked big celebrations in the ground and city. It looked as if we would have to settle for second place because Brighton were four points ahead with two matches to go. We won our last two, beating Cardiff 2-0 away and Barnsley 3-0 at home on 7 May. DeAndre Yedlin had a great match that day, racing up and down the right wing.

Football being the unpredictable sport that it is, Brighton only managed to get one more point in their last two matches, so we finished top. We had Jack Grealish scoring ten-man Villa's equaliser in the dying moments of their match against the Seagulls to thank for that. We finished on 94 points, eight fewer than the previous promotion season of 2009/10 but it felt just as good. We had a spontaneous party after the Barnsley match. It wasn't planned that way, but the lads were elated at the last-minute title win. Someone started playing music in the dressing room, we partied there, then we all went to the players' lounge. Other members of staff appeared when they heard the noise we were making. Bottles of booze kept appearing, Rafa popped in and we stayed in there for hours.

* * *

During the summer break, *more* terrible news came through: Cheick had died. During training in Beijing, he'd collapsed and they'd been unable to resuscitate him. He died on 5 June 2017, aged 30. I'd been close to Cheick, especially following our trip to Ghana. He was so loved and respected in his home country, Ivory Coast, that he was awarded the honour of a military funeral in Abidjan, attended by their prime minister.

* * *

Despite being promoted, Ashley didn't allow Rafa to be extravagant with his purchases for the new season. We signed Christian Atsu on a long-term contract and brought in Jacob Murphy and Florian Lejeune. Yoan Gouffran, Sammy Ameobi and Tim Krul moved on. We started okay but then running up to the New Year we only picked up five points from a possible 36. Starting 2018 we were in 16th place, one point off the drop zone. The lads were trying hard enough, but the modern Premier League is such a tough competition to succeed in. Rafa was becoming frustrated at not being allowed to bring in new players to the squad. He was able to bring in goalkeeper Martin Dúbravka on loan, though.

Our first match of the year was a good 1-0 away win at Stoke. Christian Atsu and Ayoze Pérez were a handful for them and the back four kept it tight. We completed a four-match winning streak against Arsenal at home in April. The lads fought back from 1-0 down to win 2-1 when Matt Ritchie scored midway through the second half against a tidy opposition, putting us on 41 points with five matches remaining, assuring safety. We needed that cushion, because we then lost the next four, but ended the season with a great display against Chelsea at home, winning 3-0, meaning we finished in tenth place.

* * *

As a manager, Rafa was great. He was always supportive of his medical staff. He undoubtedly loves football. We had a running joke about being, 'Rafa'd'. If you bumped into him about six o'clock in the evening, as he was leaving the training ground, and spoke to him ... and if he was in the right mood, he would start a conversation. Before you knew it, he would be regaling you about football, be it at Liverpool, Inter or Real Madrid. Highly entertaining and fascinating but you knew you wouldn't be getting home until past seven! It was during one of these chats, being Rafa'd, that he told me he'd been offered a fortune to go to China but had turned them down because he was determined to win a trophy for our fans.

* * *

Before the start of 2018/19, Rafa was publicly vocal about the need to bring in new players. Ashley didn't respond to those requests, but Martin Dúbravka did sign a long-term contract and Fabian Schär signed from Deportivo. In a lot of ways, this season was like the previous campaign. We didn't start well, going the first ten matches without a win and gaining only three points, but then we picked up points here and there. Rafa was awarded the manager of the month award for November, but in January we lost 2-0 at home to Man Utd, then 2-1 away to Chelsea, putting us third from bottom. Rafa signed Miguel Almirón from Atlanta United. The addition of Miggy helped us pick up positive results. He linked up well with Ayoze, who had formed a good partnership up front with Salomón Rondón.

On 9 March we played Everton at home. By half-time they were 2-0 up, despite our lads not playing too badly. The second half was different. We put them under pressure but didn't pull one back until midway through the half. We scored twice in the last ten minutes to take a well-deserved victory. Ayoze was great that match. Their keeper, Jordan Pickford, took a lot of criticism for allowing his passion as a Sunderland supporter to get the better of him. The Toon fans loved it! We were in 13th place after that win and it stayed that way until the end of the season, when we had an impressive 4-0 victory away to Fulham.

We had our suspicions that Rafa was going to go, especially when once again he stated that he would only stay if Ashley provided him with the funds to build the team he required. Even the promise of Joelinton wasn't enough to keep Rafa. The club announced that it would not be renewing his contract; when it expired one week later, on 30 June, Rafa was gone. Next, Ashley sold Ayoze Pérez to Leicester.

On 17 July the club announced that Steve Bruce was to be the next manager. The response from the fans was mixed, but some were immediately hostile. It was obviously nice to have a local lad who knows the area, but many felt he wouldn't achieve the success that Rafa had. His time at Sunderland didn't help at all with some of the fans, who were very vocal in their dissent to his appointment. For many long-term supporters that was the final straw, and they didn't renew their season tickets, citing the sale of Ayoze as well as what they considered to be a manager downgrade. Not a great situation for Steve to be walking into.

Chapter 23

Steve Bruce

STEVE BRUCE did his best to acknowledge the achievements of Rafa and he asked for a bit of time from the fans so that he could get established. He was full of enthusiasm for the task of reviving his hometown club. He joined us when we were on pre-season training in China. He introduced us to his coaches, Stephen Clemence and Steve Agnew. I already knew the new manager, having met him while the team was away in Malaysia with Bobby Robson playing in the 2003/04 pre-season Asia Cup. Birmingham City were staying in the same Kuala Lumpur hotel, so having that connection was a bonus. With the medical staff, he gave us his full support and was always respectful of our decisions. I found him to be an honest and kind manager. From day one, however, he had an uphill task persuading some of the fans that he was the right man. History has shown that the Toon managers who start off with this difficult task are alright until there's a run of bad results. He later admitted that several previous managers had contacted him to warn him how difficult the job would be.

The stadium wasn't full for our first match of 2019/20, at home to Arsenal. We lost 1-0 in a tight affair. On our third outing we picked up our first points in a win away at Spurs, in our orange strip. We absorbed a lot of pressure but, from a great move from the back, Christian Atsu crossed the ball to Joelinton on the right side of the box. Joe seemed to have acres of space and knocked the ball neatly into the bottom left corner to get his first goal for the club. Hopes were raised, but after that we drifted down the table and things weren't so great when we lost 5-0 away to Leicester in a match that Ayoze Pérez was playing for the opposition. A consolation to that hammering was a home win against Man Utd the following week, at the beginning of October. That lifted us out of the bottom three into the mid-table bunch.

We had our ups and downs after that. On 7 March we beat Southampton away, leaving us in 13th on 35 points ... The season stopped ... The SARS-CoV-2 virus had reached the UK. Although the cases took a bit longer to increase in the North East, Covid was starting to cause problems and the government was hell-bent on introducing the measures it did, meaning we were all in lockdown. At first we thought it would only be for two weeks or so, to 'flatten the curve', but the government then extended it and, before you knew it, we were at the time of the season when we should be winding down and watching the FA Cup Final, but everything was still on hold.

It was at this time that a rumour started about interest from Saudi Arabia in buying the club. Shortly after this it was reported that something called the 'PIF' had made a bid of £300m, which the English Premier League (EPL) were assessing. We presumed that Ashley had accepted the bid, but it had to be agreed by the EPL. This started lots of speculation among the fans. Almost everyone I spoke to was for the move. There were people in the media, nearly all of them not linked in any way to NUFC, who objected to the purchase for various reasons. These included human rights, a pirate and illegal TV streaming service in Saudi, and something called 'sportswashing' (sponsoring a team or event to exploit people's love of sport to 'wash' their stained image clean). The EPL said, to paraphrase, that the fans were not to worry about the suitability of prospective buyers, because that was what the 'Owners' and Directors' Test' was for.

At the beginning of June we were told the epidemic was under control and restrictions were being gradually lifted. We were still in the FA Cup, through to the sixth round. We played Man City in an empty St James' Park under the revised Covid rules. It was so good to be out of lockdown and involved in a game of football. In fact, it was a *massive relief.* Watching the match, it was hard not to get the impression it was a training match with the players' voices echoing around the cavernous stadium. The lads played well, but Man City had a very good team against us that day and we lost 2-0. In the league, there were still nine matches left and they packed them into a five-week period from 21 June to 26 July. It wasn't a great spell for results: we managed two wins, three draws and lost four. It was enough to be safe. The last match was at home to champions Liverpool. Dwight Gayle scored for us after 24 seconds, but we went down 3-1 and finished in 13th place, ten points above the drop zone on 44 points.

* * *

Before the start of the new season, there was once again talk of the takeover. We saw that the prospective buyers were fronted by Amanda Staveley, of PCP Capital Partners. Amanda's father had created the Lightwater Valley Adventure Park, near Ripon, on land that his family had owned since the 16th century. For a while she'd co-owned the park with her brother.

The group interested in purchasing the club was a consortium. Amanda's company, which included her husband Mehrdad Ghodoussi, potentially would have a 10 per cent share in NUFC.

RB Sports & Media (the Reuben family) would also own 10 per cent. The majority backing (80 per cent) would come from the mysterious PIF (Public Investment Fund) of Saudi Arabia, which as far as we could tell was their royal family's sovereign wealth fund, including the crown prince himself, Mohammed bin Salman. The constant talk couldn't have been easy for Steve Bruce, especially as most people were expecting him to be sacked if they bought Ashley out.

At the beginning of August, depressing news came out that the PIF had withdrawn their bid, citing the prolonged process and uncertainties with Covid. Well, that was that for another year or so, we thought. Yet another false dawn with regards to the sale of the club. Many fans were extremely frustrated by the on-off news.

Stoke City came to Newcastle for our final pre-season friendly. Their manager was Michael O'Neill. He told Steve Bruce the story about the time I 'saved his life'. Of course, it wasn't that dramatic but it was pretty scary at the time. Jim Smith was manager and we'd been away touring in the south of Sweden, playing matches before the start of the 1989/90 season. It was our last night and we were in a nightclub. Someone had dropped and smashed a glass. Michael slipped on the wet floor, cutting his wrist on the broken glass. He severed his ulnar artery and there was blood spurting all over the place. It was a right panic. I grabbed something and pressed on the wound as hard as I could. I've never sobered up so quickly! I then had to spend the rest of the night trying to get some sleep in a Swedish A&E department while they fixed Michael's artery. That's the sort of things football physios end up doing. Shortly after that, Michael left the club and signed for Dundee United.

* * *

The 2020/21 season started late, in September. The manager brought in Callum Wilson and Ryan Fraser from Bournemouth. Joe Willock came in on loan until the end of the season. The start was mixed, getting a repeating win, loss and draw combination in the first six matches. In December we started a nine-match run without a win and picked up only two points. The last of these outings was a 2-1 defeat at home to Leeds. To say the fans were getting restless once again is an understatement. There was a lot of anger.

It was at this time that my friend DeAndre Yedlin left to go and play in Turkey. I would miss DeAndre about the place. It was unusual to work with American players and he had an interesting background. A bit like John Barnes, he liked to engage in conversations about things such as culture, race and religion, which is unusual for footballers. He would sometimes come to training wearing the most outrageous outfits. I started off asking him where he bought them from, 'cos I'd like to get some for myself', which he didn't like the sound of. He eventually realised I was taking the mickey.

After the turn of the year Graeme Jones arrived from Bournemouth to assist Steve Bruce as a coach. Graeme was a very charismatic lad and immediately had a good rapport with the players. He's from Gateshead originally, so that Geordie pedigree always helps, of course. There seemed a slightly strange dynamic among the coaches and manager then, though. It was difficult to put your finger on it.

At the end of January we had a good 2-0 win away at Everton, against expectations. We then had a run of nine matches when we only managed one win and four draws. One of those draws was at home to Wolves towards the end of February. We'd gone 1-0 up at the start of the second half when Jamaal Lascelles scored a great header from Ryan Fraser's cross. Miggy and Allan Saint-Maximin were in sparkling form for us. Midway through the half, Steve brought off Emil Krafth and replaced him with Matt Ritchie. Immediately after the substitution, Wolves equalised from a cross and header. Another two points dropped. We were three points above the drop zone. Steve Bruce had another falling-out with the local newspapers after this and any media interviews from then on became very tense affairs.

* * *

On Sunday, 28 February I heard the terrible news that Glenn Roeder had died. He'd been treated in 2003 for a brain tumour while he was managing West Ham. By the time he was promoted to the manager's position at Newcastle in 2006, we thought he was cured. Indeed, he survived for 18 years after the diagnosis, but he finally left us at the age of 65. He was such a lovely man, and a great friend. It was around this time that I was starting to think about my future. I'd finally made the decision to retire, ideally in two years' time. This decision had taken a lot of soul-searching, as football was a massive part of my life. I'd become obsessed with this decision for a while, and I found myself talking about it all the time, which was a mistake.

* * *

The last of a run of seven matches without a win was a 2-2 draw at home to Spurs at the beginning of April, when Joe Willock got us the equaliser in the last five minutes. We were in 17th position on 29 points. League safety came when we travelled to Leicester and got a great 4-2 win. We were 4-0 up, but they scored two late goals and made us sweat it out. Martin Dúbravka saved twice from Ayoze Pérez to keep us from disaster and basically assured that we would be in the Premier League for another season. We were kept waiting for mathematical certainty when we lost at home 4-3 to Man City in an end-to-end match. The lead switched four times, but they won, helped by a Torres hat-trick. The eventual champions controlled the last 20 minutes, leaving everyone watching very frustrated on the night. We went on to win our last two matches and finished in 12th place on 45 points, a slight improvement on the previous season, but higher than we'd dared to hope for most of the season.

* * *

The next campaign started badly; we had to wait until match 15 in December for a win. But ... I'm getting ahead of myself here because a *lot* had happened since the season had got underway. Steve was still in charge at the start of the season on 15 August. However, away from the pitch, Newcastle supporters had started a public campaign to question the tactics of the EPL in stonewalling the purchase of the club, despite the PIF consortium reportedly withdrawing their bid. The Newcastle United Supporters Trust, or NUST, played a vital role in the fans' activism. They created a petition that received 110,000 signatures. The Independent Football Ombudsman and dozens of MPs wrote on behalf of supporters to Richard Masters (Chief Executive Officer of the EPL). Further pressure came when Prime Minister Boris Johnson said the EPL had to explain the reason for the delay in the decision of the Owners' and Directors' Test.

Against this backdrop we lost the first match, at home, to West Ham. We were in the lead twice and were ahead after the break. They levelled, and then about an hour in they scored twice in three minutes and knocked the stuffing out of the team and the crowd. Next, we were away to Villa. That match down in Birmingham was the first time our fans had been able to travel for nearly 18 months. We took 3,000 excited supporters down but, despite a spirited performance, we lost 2-0.

* * *

The takeover rumour mill and media reports went into overdrive in September. The club accused the EPL of officially rejecting the consortium's bid; the EPL responded by saying they hadn't rejected it. By now the club had taken legal arbitration action and had filed a separate claim through the UK Competition Appeal Tribunal (CAT). There was a lot of interest generated among the Geordie public and 33,000 people watched an online CAT hearing. I think most people assumed the legal arguments would go on for months if not years. The EPL had been accused of 'following the money', because they were allegedly being lobbied by the Qatari-based sports-streaming channel beIN Sports to block the purchase. To summarise, the issue seemed to not really be about human rights, but about the Saudi government's diplomatic spat with Qatar over television rights. The Saudis were blocking Qatari beIN Sports satellite transmissions in their kingdom, instead promoting a pirate entity called beoutQ that was transmitting beIN content. The EPL was making hundreds of millions of pounds in TV rights from beIN, so let's say they at least had an obligation to listen to beIN's gripe with the Saudis. All very complicated for people like me who take no interest in this sort of thing, but nevertheless it's necessary to acknowledge what was going on.

On 2 October we were down in the Black Country playing Wolves. We'd drawn our previous two matches, including doing well down at Watford to get a draw in the previous outing. It drizzled all game at Molineux. After a slow start they went ahead then hit the bar. Allan Saint-Maximin did his stuff and created enough chaos in their box for a rebound to come out to Jeff Hendrick, who drilled the ball into the net to equalise. It wasn't to be our day, though, when Hwang Hee-chan scored his second goal on the hour to give them a 2-1 win. That was the cue for our away support to vent their anger with the club. There was constant talk now from the fans, saying they wanted Steve out. Undoubtedly his days were numbered if he didn't start getting some victories.

On 6 October, news emerged that Saudi Arabia had lifted their ban on the broadcasting of beIN Sports in their country. Perhaps those who were closely studying what was going on with the takeover knew this was an important development, but had I known about it, it would have meant nothing to me.

Sometimes, things happen slowly and then very quickly. The following day it was officially announced that Mike Ashley had finally sold the football club to the consortium (Saudi beIN ban lifted, PIF consortium immediately passes the EPL Owners' and Directors' Test ... club sold). Images started popping on the news of groups of teenage lads outside St James' Park wearing their mams' checked tea towels on their heads fastened on with bootlaces. Before long, hundreds had turned out for one of those memorable moments in the club's history. I had no idea whether Steve would be kept on. He had a good nucleus of a team with the likes of Allan Saint-Maximin, Miggy Almerón, Joelinton and Callum Wilson. I hoped with the right financial support he could do well. I don't believe many others thought that. One of the first things Amanda Staveley said was that Steve's job was safe ... for now.

The next match was home to Spurs. It was Steve Bruce's 1000th match in all competitions as a manager. There was tremendous excitement in the city. We were all well up for it, with Mike Ashley a memory and the new owners making all the right noises. What a scene the Wor Flags display made before kick-off. Callum scored within a couple of minutes of the start; the stadium erupted in a tumult of deafening noise and thousands of flashes of black-and-white flags surrounding the pitch whirled frantically, bringing back memories of the glory days.

But, it wasn't to be the result we all wanted. By half-time we were 3-1 down. We managed to get it back to 3-2 at the death but it was too late to get an equaliser. Spurs had the lion's share of the possession, which added to the frustration. The honeymoon for the manager was immediately over and many fans once again expressed their disdain for him, hurling abuse before and during the match. In the second half it was brutal. That was to be his last match in charge. On 20 October it was announced that he'd gone. I think Steve saw the writing on the wall in fluorescent neon block capitals and negotiated his exit with the new owners. Graeme Jones took over as interim manager. Eddie Howe was announced as the next manager on 8 November. We were in 19th place, on five points and winless.

Chapter 24

Eddie Howe

EDDIE'S FIRST match in charge was at St James', against Brentford. Before that we got to watch Eddie take training. He's a manager who likes to be actively involved, leading the training. His coaching reminded me a bit of Bobby Robson, when he first started down at the Riverside at Chester-le-Street. Eddie's style was very impressive. He organised drills and games that revolved around speed of play and speed of thought. We saw some of that straightaway in the home match against Brentford, although Eddie had to stay away because he had Covid. We took the lead through Jamaal Lascelles's header, but they equalised immediately. Then they went ahead before Joelinton equalised near the end of the first half. They took the lead on an hour, but we salvaged a draw when Allan Saint-Maximin played a lovely pass to Ryan Fraser, then received his cross back with a volley into the bottom left corner, before doing a cartwheel and tumble. It ended 3-3. What a breathless start!

Despite being bottom on six points, the city was buzzing again. We waited another three matches after that for a win. First, we lost away to Arsenal, but competed well. Next, we drew at home to fellow strugglers Norwich after Ciaran Clark was sent off after only ten minutes. The win came in early December, home to

Burnley. Callum scored a good centre-forward's goal when Nick Pope (playing for Burnley at the time) dropped the ball and the forward gave himself enough space to bury it in the net. We had a hard run of matches after that, and the results proved it. We lost away to Leicester and Liverpool, then 4-0 at home to Man City before getting a draw at home to Man Utd just before the New Year. The lads did impress that match, Allan scoring a lovely goal in the first ten minutes, cutting inside then hitting the shot into the top right corner. Both teams had chances after that but they equalised when Cavani's rebounded shot came straight back to him to pass into the net. Right at the end Jacob Murphy hit the post, Miggy picked up the rebound and it was heading for the top left corner only for De Gea to make a fingertip save. Just a draw, but we knew the team had turned a corner.

We started 2022 in a terrible league position but with plenty of optimism. Eddie signed Kieran Trippier from Atlético Madrid, so we all expected a victory at home to League One Cambridge United in the FA Cup third round. It's a match that the 5,000 travelling Cambridge fans will never forget, and Kieran probably won't either: we lost 1-0. That result aside, the city's confidence in the new owners and manager was reflected in the following results, winning six and getting two draws from the next eight matches. New signing Bruno Guimarães made his debut against Everton during that run, on 8 January, in a 3-1 win. His presence made a difference to the team. Twenty points is about half the total needed for safety and that run proved to be the turning point for us.

We were shocked to hear on 20 February that Steve Black had died at the age of 64. He had one or two health issues while he was with us under McClaren, but I was completely taken aback when I heard the news. Blackie really was an amazing coach, blazing a trail before his time. More importantly, he was a unique person, and that's why he had such a lasting effect on the people he met. A proper, proud Geordie.

On 13 March we lost away to Chelsea, ending our good run. We then lost the next two, also away from home, but victory in the home match against Wolves heralded a run of four wins on the trot. When we won that fourth match, 3-0 away to Norwich, that put us in ninth place on 43 points. Liverpool pegged our egos back when they beat us 1-0 at home, going top. Next, Man City rubbed salt in our wounds, beating us 5-0 in a masterclass that then put *them* top. We steadied the ship with a solid 2-0 victory over Arsenal in our last home match of the season. Bruno showed some real class in midfield. We rounded off the season with an away win at Burnley, which unfortunately relegated them but meant we finished a respectable 11th.

Over the close season, I had some to-and-fro with the HR department. They were aware of my decision to retire. The original plan was that my colleague James Haycock would work alongside me as head physio, then take over my role. However, he was offered the position as chief physiotherapist at Crystal Palace, which he accepted. That left a tricky situation for the club; they had to plan for a new head physio, because they knew I wanted to leave. They began the search for my replacement, so although I would have preferred one more year, I decided that the best thing I could do was to agree an immediate leaving date, and so be it. After four decades I was no longer the Toon physio.

I didn't take part in pre-season training for the first time in 40 years but Eddie and Jason Tindall were very gracious in inviting me to come in to say my goodbyes to the lads. So often in football that's not possible, so I'm grateful to them for that. The club bosses were also very kind in inviting my family and me to the opening match of the season, when we were in the directors' box (a first for me!) to watch a comfortable 2-0 win against Nottingham Forest to get the season started, on 6 August 2022. I was also presented with a signed shirt at half-time. I was asked to come down to the dressing room after the match, when the lads presented me with a leaving present.

Things are a lot different from when I started. Then there was one physio for all players from the youth team, through reserves and first team. There was one kit manager and a couple of ladies to do the laundry. The managers might have had an assistant and a couple of coaches. Eddie Howe has undoubtedly raised the bar in coaching and management standards. He often puts in 12-hour days at the training ground. He runs the training sessions. His attention to detail is remarkable. To help him with this, he has six coaches, four strength and conditioning coaches, eight analysts and a nutritionist. On the medical side there's a sports physician, six physios and four masseurs (solely for the senior squad). There has been some turnover at senior physio level since I left. That's football for you. The kit manager Tommo has four assistants and four laundry staff. The club brought in a sporting director, Dan Ashworth, who was the FA's former Director of Elite Development and after that had helped to transform Brighton. Shortly after Dan came in, Darren Eales was appointed as CEO. He had a background in law and economics and had been CEO of Atlanta United FC in the States.

When my retirement news got out, I was overwhelmed by the response. My younger two sons, Ben and James, were forever coming to show me their phones with kind messages from past and present players, managers and coaches on Twitter. I was very humbled.

There's a phenomenon after retirement called 'OMY': 'One More Year'. I hadn't quit just yet. I still have my private clinic on

Osborne Avenue in Jesmond, which kept me going. And then Hartlepool United needed some help, so I covered their training sessions for the start of the 2022/23 season and helped find them a permanent physio. I then travelled to the United Arab Emirates to do some work with Al Ain FC in the UAE Pro League. I felt the need to do one more year (OMY!) to get the financial security for my family. Or that's what I said to myself as an excuse! My eldest son, Jonathan, has lived and worked in Dubai and Abu Dhabi for about ten years, so it was nice to spend some time with him and his girlfriend, Olga. Unfortunately, that job didn't work out as planned, so I returned to Newcastle after several months.

* * *

On 6 February 2023, in the early hours of the morning, a massive earthquake struck southern Turkey and north-western Syria. Close to 60,000 unfortunate souls lost their lives. One of them was Christian Atsu. Christian was at this time playing for Hatayspor in Turkey. At first, we didn't know that he'd been involved, but was missing. Part of the Hatayspor's headquarters in Antakya had collapsed. Then came the sad news that his body had been found on 18 February. He was 31 years old. He had a state funeral ceremony in Accra attended by the Ghana president and Chris Hughton, who had just been promoted to be their national team coach. Bless him. I've known so many men in football who have died too soon. This book can attest to that.

Of course, I had to go to Wembley to watch the 2023 EFL Cup Final on 26 February. The Metropolitan Police estimated that there were 100,000 Geordies in London for the final, with and without tickets. What a show the fans put on in Trafalgar Square the night before. It has become a firm tradition of the Toon supporters to take over that part of London whenever we have a final, and long may it continue. Of course, it wasn't to be; yet another Wembley final defeat. What more do you expect? As a consolation, two weeks after that I was presented with the Bob Cass Award at the North East Football Writers' Association Awards on 13 March. It was very unexpected, but such an honour. It was painful to watch the short video they made of my time at the club, especially a recording of an interview I did shortly after arriving there, when for some inexplicable reason I sounded like a narrator using received English on a 1950's Pathé newsreel!

* * *

Well, overall, I think things are changing at the Toon. We have a talented team, great manager and committed owners. It's only a matter of time now until we start winning … isn't it? We need to reach our rightful place in the top six clubs in England. The fans have always been the best, so it's about time the club caught up to match them. We got off to a flying start, finishing 2022/23 season in fourth place, qualifying for the Champion's League. Most of 2023/24 was a little bit disappointing, if we're being honest. We went out of all cup competitions and failed to grab a Champions League place, but at the end we had the excitement of competing for the Europa League spot. The manager didn't have it easy with regards to injuries. However, the head of rehabilitation, Sean Beech, is a very bright and capable physio and I know he'll get it right working alongside the doc, Paul Catterson, and Dan Hodges the head of performance.

I'm looking forward to spending more time with my younger two boys, Ben and James. They're both still at school in Morpeth and play football for Ponteland Juniors. There's still time for them to 'make the grade'. Of course, I must thank my wife, Helen, who has held everything together all these years.

I couldn't bring myself to watch the *We Are Newcastle United* series on Amazon Prime; I miss the crack too much. I've heard it was very good. The owners appear to 'get' what being a Newcastle supporter and a Geordie is all about. I hope they do. If they understand what it feels like to see the city skyline appear when your train from London rounds the bend in Gateshead with the majestic Tyne Bridge in all her glory spanning *our* river, then perhaps they know.

Postscript

I WANT to dedicate this book to my parents, Pat and Derek. Dad died after we'd completed the first draft of the book. I decided to leave the comments about him as they'd been written. He died suddenly in the evening on Armistice Day, 11 November 2023, which is fitting for an old soldier. In the morning he went to the Metro Centre with our mother, something they did every Saturday. At 11am, Mam was in Boots at the self-service tills. She stopped doing her purchase during the two-minute silence, as did the other customers. The lime-green LED displays of the tills were flashing 'please complete your purchase, please complete your purchase'. Mam looked outside; Dad was standing to attention. She watched as those sitting beside him followed his lead and did the same. I hope you enjoy the book, Dad.

Acknowledgements

I WOULD like to thank my brother John for his hard work and dedication over the past year.

Thank you to Ian Horrocks for his support, advice, and contribution of photographs.

Thanks also to Serena Taylor and Mark Hannen of NUFC for their contribution of photographs.

Thank you to Paul Joannou, NUFC club historian, for his guidance and advice.

A sincere thank you to my friends and colleagues Kevin Keegan, Alan Shearer, Stuart Pearce, Ray Thompson and Paul Ferris for their help and contribution.

I would also like to thank the team at Pitch Publishing for their support.

Thanks also to Howard Tait for his help and ideas. And finally, a big thank you to my wife Helen for her love and patience, and to my three boys Jonathan, Benjamin and James.

Bibliography

Barton, Joey: *Joey Barton, No Nonsense* (Simon & Schuster UK Ltd, 2017)

Bellamy, Craig: *Craig Bellamy: GoodFella* (Sport Media, 2014)

Black, Steve: *Blackie: The Steve Black Story* (Mainstream Publishing, 2005)

Chaplin, Michael: *Newcastle United Stole My Heart* (C. Hurst & Co. Ltd, 2021)

Dalglish, Kenny: *Dalglish, My Autobiography* (Hodder & Stoughton, 1996)

Dyer, Kieron: *Old Too Soon, Smart Too Late* (Headline Publishing Group, 2018)

Ferris, Paul: *The Boy on the Shed* (Hodder & Stoughton, 2018)

Ferris, Paul: *The Magic in the Tin* (Bloomsbury Publishing Plc, 2022)

Gascoigne, Paul: *Gazza, My Story* (Headline Book Publishing, 2004)

Ginola, David: *David Ginola: Le Magnifique* (CollinsWillow, 2000)

Hardy, Martin: *Touching Distance* (deCoubertin Books Ltd, 2015)

Hardy, Martin: *Tunnel of Love* (deCoubertin Books Ltd, 2017)

Hutchinson, Roger: *The Toon* (Mainstream Publishing Co. Ltd, 1997)

Jackson, Dan: *The Northumbrians* (C. Hurst & Co. Ltd, 2019)

Keegan, Kevin: *Kevin Keegan, My Life in Football* (Macmillan, 2018)

Keegan, Kevin: *My Autobiography* (Little, Brown and Company, 1997)

Macdonald, Malcolm: *Win!* (Pelham Books, 1997)

Robson, Sir Bobby: *Sir Bobby Robson, Living the Game* (Weidenfeld & Nicolson, 2003)

Shearer, Alan: *Alan Shearer, My Story So Far* (Hodder & Stoughton, 1998)

Walker, Ray: *The Ultimate Newcastle United Trivia Book* (HRP House, 2021)